"Drs. Pieniadz and Young-Eisendrath are on the pioneering edge with their elegant and highly effective model of Dialogue Therapy and Real Dialogue. As someone who has worked for years to help heal the broken-hearted, and offer hope to those who steadfastly believe in love despite their many bumps and bruises along the way, I'm thrilled to discover this graceful, heartfelt, compellingly simple, yet brilliantly deep work to awaken our ability to grow greater levels of compassion and care between us. These two superb luminaries are my new relationship gurus."

—**Katherine Woodward Thomas, M.A., MFT,**
New York Times bestselling author of
*Conscious Uncoupling: 5 Steps to Living
Happily Even After*

"This ambitious, beautifully written text represents decades of accumulated clinical wisdom. Integrating feminism, Buddhism, psychoanalysis, and empirical scholarship, the authors show how to help antagonistic parties to listen respectfully, grow in self-knowledge and autonomy, and appreciate the equal humanity of the other. Their work is both inspiring and quintessentially practical. I recommend this book to all therapists who work with couples as well as to professionals in the fields of coaching, consulting, and conflict resolution."

—**Nancy McWilliams, Ph.D.,**
author of *Psychoanalytic Diagnosis* and
Psychoanalytic Psychotherapy

Dialogue Therapy for Couples and Real Dialogue for Opposing Sides

A clear, cogent, and comprehensive account of the rationale and methods of Dialogue Therapy and Real Dialogue, this volume introduces models of facilitated dialogue designed specifically to end polarization.

This book offers a straightforward and comprehensive encounter with some of the most effective theories and methods to facilitate dialogue and disrupt deadening power struggles between life partners, grown children and parents, siblings, co-workers, and others whose conflicts have led to harmful polarizations. The book is based on ideas and relational models from mindfulness and psychoanalysis that have not been applied in this unique way before. This melding of mindfulness (containment, concentration, equanimity, maintaining a "mindful gap") with the psychoanalytic understanding of projection and projective identification (the "hijacking" of our subjective experiences) creates much more than light at the end of the tunnel. It engenders the acceptance of another that leads to love and insight, based on the recognition and acknowledgement of our autonomy and our common humanity in the midst of conflict.

This book introduces a new, revolutionary model for couple therapists, life coaches, group facilitators, and leaders to open a mindful space that increases witnessing capacities in the midst of emotional conflict without imposing goals of agreement, reconciliation, or compromise.

Jean Pieniadz, Ph.D., is a psychologist, psychoanalyst, and supervisor in private practice. She is a founding and current faculty and board member of the Vermont Institute for the Psychotherapies. Her publications are in the areas of developmental psychology, feminist ethics, and neuropsychology.

Polly Young-Eisendrath, Ph.D., is a psychologist, writer, speaker, and Jungian analyst. She has published eighteen books (translated into twenty languages), including *The Self-Esteem Trap* and *Love Between Equals*. A lifelong Buddhist practitioner, she is also a mindfulness teacher. Her podcast is "Enemies: From War to Wisdom" (www.young-eisendrath.com).

Dialogue Therapy for Couples and Real Dialogue for Opposing Sides

Methods Based on Psychoanalysis and Mindfulness

Jean Pieniadz and
Polly Young-Eisendrath

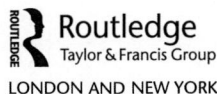
Routledge
Taylor & Francis Group

LONDON AND NEW YORK

First published 2022
by Routledge
2 Park Square, Milton Park, Abingdon, Oxon OX14 4RN

and by Routledge
605 Third Avenue, New York, NY 10158

Routledge is an imprint of the Taylor & Francis Group, an informa business

© 2022 Jean Pieniadz and Polly Young-Eisendrath

The right of Jean Pieniadz and Polly Young-Eisendrath to be identified as authors of this work has been asserted by them in accordance with sections 77 and 78 of the Copyright, Designs and Patents Act 1988.

British Library Cataloguing-in-Publication Data
A catalogue record for this book is available from the British Library

Library of Congress Cataloging-in-Publication Data
A catalog record for this book has been requested

ISBN: 978-1-032-06135-1 (hbk)
ISBN: 978-1-032-04075-2 (pbk)
ISBN: 978-1-003-20084-0 (ebk)

DOI: 10.4324/9781003200840

Typeset in Bembo
by Apex CoVantage, LLC

I dedicate this book to Joel Shapiro, with boundless love.

– JP

This book is dedicated to those who have entered into, learned, practiced, and developed Dialogue Therapy and Real Dialogue.

– PYE

Contents

Acknowledgements

I am deeply grateful for the friendship and collegiality of Dr. Polly Young-Eisendrath, who has been a great source of inspiration, support, and knowledge for me, over many years. She has been a trusted supervisor, then consultant, mentor, and co-therapist. She brings boundless energy, steadfast commitment, and confident wisdom to her every project. She is a rare gem in this wild and wonderful field of psychotherapy, and I treasure her.

My heartfelt gratitude goes out to:

The couples with whom I've worked – they have taught me so much over the years, about all the different ways to *be* a couple. I have been challenged, touched, schooled, and honored to be involved in this work with them.

My colleagues at Mansfield Psychotherapy Associates (Dan Brown, Aleta Vail, Elizabeth Goldstein, Jessica Houser, and Joel Shapiro), my peer consultation group (Debra, Brooke, and Elizabeth S.), and my psychologist friends: Joyce Pfennig, Ene Piirak, Susan Boulware, Christiane Gariépy-Boutin, who, with their unwavering friendship and support, have dialogued, joked, and creatively riffed with me about many professional experiences and ideas for several decades.

All my teachers and supervisors, in Boston, Burlington (VT), Montreal, and New York who have introduced me to writers, ideas, and sparkling bits of clinical wisdom – and shared their vulnerabilities and imperfections with such great generosity and dignity. It is all now an integral part of me.

Alana, who has always been kind, patient, curious, engaged, and an incredible fount of humor and playfulness during her mother's studies, work, and various projects. Our love is queen.

Joel Shapiro, my partner and long-standing co-therapist, who truly and deeply knows how to be in a loving partnership. He has been my relationship North Star for over forty years, an embodiment of all the values of Dialogue.

Jean Pieniadz, Ph.D.
Psychologist/Psychoanalyst

★★★

First, my co-author Jean Pieniadz was bold, brave, and intelligent every step of the way in this co-writing process. Writing a book jointly has many of the challenges a couple relationship does, and Jeannie was willing to engage with me completely and wrestle through, as needed, our own Real Dialogue for opposing sides. Also, I found Jeannie's writing and turns of phrase to be inspiring and congenial for my own style. Our work together over the decades as co-therapists and co-teachers, and in many other roles – in addition to being close friends – has made this joint venture a true pleasure. Thank you, Jeannie!

Second, my partner Robert Caper has been instrumental in clarifying my ideas and approaches to projective identification. Without his steadfast help, I would have strayed into the vague emotional landscape of less-than-complete descriptions of what happens between individuals in projective identification. His editorial and conversational help has been invaluable. Robert, your editorial incisiveness and clinical perspectives are always deeply appreciated, even when I don't say so.

Third, of course, I would not have created or practiced Dialogue Therapy without my late husband Ed Epstein. Because he trained in both socio-drama and psychodrama, as a family therapist before we met, he taught me how to bring experiential and dramatic set-ups, and interventions, into couple therapy. His imprint on Dialogue Therapy will never fade.

And fourth, both Jeannie and I want to sing the praises of our generous and witty personal editor, Frank Smecker. With his own background in psychoanalytic theory and English literature, Frank was an ideal editorial assistant: he was conscientious, thorough, and inspired, and queried us in all the right ways. He was even willing to engage Jeannie and me about the "important" usage distinctions between the words *individual* and *person*. We could not have found anyone better suited to help us with this manuscript – which he did by editing, formatting, designing, and working on the scholarship and citations. A deep bow of gratitude to you, Frank.

I won't go into elaborate detail about my Buddhist teachers (I have done so in other books, especially in *Love Between Equals*), but they and my psycho-analytic colleagues and fellow travelers have brought me the larger theoretical frameworks for Dialogue Therapy. Without their help, this amazing work with couples and others caught in harmful polarizations wouldn't exist.

And then, I want to thank all who have trained in and practiced Dialogue Therapy and Real Dialogue in its recent incarnation. The following people have made important contributions to this book through meeting with me on a regular basis in our weekly Ask Me Anything sessions: Susan Lillich, Sarah Brodie, Raven Bruce, Stella Marrie, Leeland Peterson, Rosa Maria Rigol, and Jeanne Plo. Additionally, Lisa Lewis and Lisa Featherstone have added their own important expertise, support, and queries in the development of Dialogue Therapy over these past several years. Many of the people who contributed to the initial training group – especially Doris Ferleger, Irene McHenry, and Beulah Trey – helped me to hammer out specifics in the solo and co-therapist models. And finally, Amber Rickert and Sherwin Watson, as members of my own family, and as extraordinary professionals themselves, have provided sharp questions, important challenges, and wonderful support through these last four years of developing Dialogue Therapy and Real Dialogue within its new frontiers. I am endlessly grateful for all of your contributions and ongoing inspiration. Please continue to support and engage in this work because we need to do it now, more than ever, in our fractured world.

My own team at Real Dialogue LLC is beyond what I deserve in dedication, competence, and inspiration. Paula Emery, Lori Roberts, and Chris Coltrane assist me in developing programs, marketing, communication, and podcasting/videotaping. Paula has become a dear friend as she has gotten to know not only me and my family, but every single person who has gone through the trainings. Paula coordinates programs, trainings, details, and designs for all that I do. Lori Roberts is an amazing graphic designer and media/communications director for me. Between Paula and Lori, my Pay Attention interviews and online classes are edited and produced. Chris Coltrane edits and produces my podcast, "Enemies: From War to Wisdom." All of these supports for learning and development in Dialogue Therapy and Real Dialogue would not exist without these people.

And last, but not least, is my co-host on the podcast, Eleanor Johnson, who is close to my heart in so many ways. As a dear friend, a fellow Dharma practitioner, a world visionary, and an everyday companion, Eleanor has been a tremendous support for this work. A deep bow and a big hug, as always, Eleanor!

I am sure that I am forgetting others who have been very important to Dialogue Therapy and Real Dialogue over the decades. Please forgive me if I have left you out. All of you have expanded and supported the work that has gone into this book. The mistakes are mine. May the work of Dialogue Therapy and Real Dialogue support human relationship in such a way as to end war and polarization!

Polly Young-Eisendrath, Ph.D.

Preface

Kind of miraculous, mysterious. I used to think of romantic relationships this way. Miraculous, that people from different subjective worlds discover each other, become fascinated with each other, and can even – sometimes! – stay together. Mysterious, how their communication is packaged, sometimes leaving people not in their relationship "bubble" to wonder: *how* and *why* did they just communicate in that particular way – a way I did not understand – but they seemed to nonetheless? They also suffer in their own particular ways sometimes, ways that are also hard to understand. Often, as a therapist, I have experienced partners' emotional pain having an impervious, "sealed off" quality to it – it can look like they have their own brand of unhappiness that no one else can fathom. They have their own seemingly unique and inscrutable brand of channeling their suffering to each other, as well.

During the thirty-five years I have been conducting couple therapy, and through my growing grasp of the concept of projective identification, a concept we will describe and use throughout this book, I have been blessedly relieved of some of my romantic wonder and puzzlement about couples. My awe and ignorance has been partly replaced by an appreciation for the liberating explanatory power of this concept. I learned about this idea and phenomenon in my graduate training and continuing training as a psychoanalyst, and it was only when I began consulting with Polly Young-Eisendrath in the late 1990s that I saw, with much greater clarity, the ways this psychological process operates in couples. Armed with an understanding of how projective identification affects partners' relating in their own distinct ways, I saw that couple therapy can bring about great and lasting change, and open the couple to a stronger, more flexible, and resilient bond – a bond that "breathes." The concept of projective identification, and its many implications and applications, created inroads to understanding couples that I had never thought possible.

Enter Dialogue Therapy, a technique developed by Polly and Ed Epstein in the early 1980s, which rests on the exploration of projective identifications in romantic partners. From that center point, Dialogue Therapy honors and emphasizes each individual's different and separate subjectivities. I found great freedom and creativity, a new intrigue with the "I and Thou" of it all. When I stand back, I suppose my relief can be reduced to the possibility that I found a sublimated Oedipal solution to being left out of the "parental marriage," but so be it. Meaningful, creative work with couples was the reward.

Once I began using Dialogue Therapy's techniques in my practice, I noticed many more ways in which couples can be helped, and, how partners' understanding of each other increases in manifold ways. This was a result of *their* using the therapeutic concepts my co-therapist(s) and I were offering them, as well as the skills they were building through the methods of Dialogue Therapy. Each couple could take their understanding and skills in whatever inventive direction they chose, fitting their particular relationship dialect. Their suffering was diminished. For me, once I began using this method there was no turning back – it was that impactful.

I now see Dialogue Therapy as a type of "subversion" (to paraphrase Dr. Laura Brown), something that can shake up many kinds of stalemates or drain the hostility out of many kinds of conflicts between any two parties. Polly and I began thinking about ways Real Dialogue, the skill set underlying Dialogue Therapy, can be applied to conflicts in conversations about politics, race, class, environment, and other socio-cultural issues. It seems to me that grandiose ambitions about "healing the world" can start at home, between you and me. If two can be in real dialogue, who knows how many more can be?

Jean Pieniadz, Ph.D.
Psychologist/Psychoanalyst

★★★

This publication brings me great pleasure. First, I am grateful to Dr. Pieniadz for her willingness to co-author. She and her husband Joel Shapiro learned the method of Dialogue Therapy (DT) from its cofounders – me and my late husband Ed Epstein. Suffice it to say, Jeannie and Joel go "way back," which makes Jeannie not only a dear friend and colleague, but also an excellent co-author and a treasured co-therapist.

Jeannie and Joel learned DT as other co-therapist teams back then did: by observing a couple go through the therapy process with me and Ed, and then working from the manual (my first book on DT) *Hags and Heroes: A Feminist Approach to Jungian Psychotherapy with Couples* (1984). After that, Ed and I supervised Jeannie and Joel, who also read my second book on DT, *You're Not What I Expected: Love After the Romance has Ended* (1993). These were the informal methods we used back then to train therapists; there was no certification process because Ed and I did not want to formalize DT's practice.

As you will see, much has happened in the world of Dialogue Therapy since the mid-1990s. In fact, DT has changed substantially even in the last decade, and so have the teachings and trainings that support it. You will read about this history in Chapter 1.

My special pleasure in having my fourth book on Dialogue Therapy published, is I believe that DT and its sibling, Real Dialogue (RD) for Opposing Sides, have grown into powerful, refined methods that can be taught and learned within the larger arena of mental health practices (in the case of DT) and adjacent arenas of coaching, facilitation, mediation, and negotiation in non-mental health professions (in the case of RD). Through continued use and practice, these methods have matured and developed within a limited circle of practitioners that has not been primarily academic, but clinical.

When Ed and I designed Dialogue Therapy and then began practicing and teaching it, we wanted to study how frameworks of equality (between the sexes) and autonomy (personal sovereignty) contribute to couple and family therapy. Borrowing from psychodrama, we created a model that combined psychoanalytic ideas and techniques with feminism so as to produce a dramatic intervention. We did not want to become a training institute, but instead wanted to change how therapists thought about and helped couples and families. We also enjoyed using this method while working with couples because it taught *us* a lot about being a couple, and we found that the same thing happened when we taught the method to other co-therapist teams, many of whom were married couples.

Consequently, we offered our Foundational Training in Dialogue Therapy as a "professional retreat" (with continuing education credits). There, therapists could learn and develop skills that they could then go on to use as they wanted, in their clinical practices, their own relationships, and with couples in therapy.

While reading the history of Dialogue Therapy, you will discover that all that has changed now. This book is the result of those changes. There are a couple nuances about the changes I want to highlight here: first, what it's been like to do this therapy for more than three decades, exclusively in a co-therapist conjoint model, and then to switch to designing, practicing, and teaching a solo model; and second, what it's been like, in these recent few years, to teach Dialogue Therapy to a broad range of mental health practitioners, and Real Dialogue to coaches and facilitators – most of whom have no particular background in psychoanalysis, psychodrama, or Jungian theory, which was what attracted trainees to this method in earlier decades.

First, I have gone through a kind of "religious" transformation myself, to admit that Dialogue Therapy can be done effectively by a *solo* therapist instead of a co-therapist team. For decades, I would say, often with religious-like fervor, that it would be *impossible* to do an effective job with this style of "short-term anxiety-provoking psychoanalytic therapy" for couples without co-therapists. The intensity and drama of the method, along with its focus on projective identification, required, so I believed, that each *partner has their own therapist*. I thought of this as a kind of inviolable law. And then, in 2016, I began teaching the method to larger general audiences. I gradually had to admit that a co-therapist conjoint model of *four adults together* for multiple meetings (that carry a steep cost for having two therapists in the room) was often not practical because it seemed too expensive and too hard to schedule. And besides, there were not many mental health professionals who could or wanted to do it.

In 2016, in Burlington, Vermont – my first weekend introduction of this new "brand of Dialogue Therapy," based especially on mindfulness and psychoanalysis – I attracted experienced and mature therapists from all over the country. They were eager to learn because they had read my earlier books about DT, but they didn't feel they could practice in a co-therapy model. I understood then that I needed to change the original model.

And so I became a solo therapist myself, doing Dialogue Therapy with couples. Of course, I also continued to practice the co-therapist model with Jeannie, but I began to systematize and develop the solo model. I also knew that Ed Epstein had used Dialogue Therapy as a solo therapist, but I had never observed him and knew that he had not systematized it for training and teaching. During these last four years, I have been developing as a solo therapist in the method, while trying to refine the teaching and training of this model. At the same time, I've been developing the overall training model and offering it in several trainings nationally and in Canada. This has been a whirlwind because I have been learning, as well as teaching, at top speed almost around the clock.

In this book, we present, compare, and contrast the co-therapist and solo models. You will learn about both, in detail. Here, I simply want to reflect that doing Dialogue Therapy with a co-therapist, especially a co-therapist who is your spouse or your professional partner, can be a true joy and pleasure, as well as a developmental challenge to your own relationship. Dialogue Therapy is dramatic, theatrical. Doing it, we learn about ourselves and our closest relationships. When I do Dialogue Therapy with my co-therapist Jean Pieniadz, I enjoy the experience even when it challenges me at every level of my being. When I do Dialogue Therapy as a solo therapist, I enjoy the *later meetings* with the couples because I witness directly their changes and skills. Being alone in the room with an embattled couple can be deeply challenging and emotionally exhausting, especially in some of the early meetings when couples begin to practice their skills in the midst of conflicts. To some extent, of course, this is the nature of couple therapy. Dialogue Therapy is especially intense and dramatic. And so having a co-therapist as your Reflecting Team (for processing and interpreting what is happening in the room) adds more than two heads: it adds mental space that may be absent for a solo therapist.

On the other side of the coin, even though I may find myself mourning the loss of my early religious fervor for the co-therapy, I am very gratified by the results of the solo model. In both my own cases and in clinical ones that I hear and teach about in my online "Ask Me Anything" group – a small group of certified professionals learning to use the solo model (although some also use the co-therapist model) – I have come to see that the solo approach to Dialogue Therapy is viable, powerful, and practical.

This brings me to the other issue: how I have developed as a trainer and teacher of this method. In 2019, I published a book about Dialogue Therapy, written for couples themselves: *Love Between Equals: Relationship as a Spiritual Path*. I wrote that book to launch this new phase of Dialogue Therapy in which it would enter a larger audience and conversation about how to relate to an equal through the process of respectful conflict, differentiation, and the growth of true love. I knew that I would then need to develop the model for teaching Dialogue Therapy to a larger professional audience.

The process of developing and teaching Dialogue Therapy, and Real Dialogue, has been the cutting edge of my own development as a therapist and human being in the last four years or so. I have learned not only to sharpen my ability to see and describe the subtle dimensions of unconscious communication via *projective identification*, but also, that difficult conversations and negotiations are *possible between strangers*, but *only* when they are structured and facilitated in such a way that the two people can *slow down* and *perceive* what each person is actually seeing, hearing, and feeling during experiences of emotional threat.

My own ability to work with projective identification, in conditions of emotional threat, has allowed me to discern how and why *mindfulness* (precisely trained awareness, within states of concentration and equanimity) must be applied in difficult conversations between adults. This kind of application is at the heart of training to be a psychoanalyst. As we face an increasingly dangerous, polarized world, we want to find ways to work with our vastly different views of reality. We recognize that to solve the problems of climate, disease, war, and racism, first we must handle our differences peacefully and wisely.

Consequently, my life, my spiritual practice, and my professional practices are now dedicated to teaching and training these kinds of specialized dialogical practices (Dialogue Therapy and Real Dialogue) as the only means I know for engaging in peaceful confrontations between people on opposing sides of important issues. I believe these forms of facilitated dialogue, which have commanded my attention since the mid-1980s, are unique in their ability to transform dangerous unconscious communication in high-risk situations. For this reason, I take great pride and pleasure in bringing out this book to further their use and development.

Polly Young-Eisendrath, Ph.D.

1 Dialogue Therapy for marriage and other relationships in the twenty-first century

Today's marriage has the goals of close relating as well as sharing tasks and decisions. Partners want to be equals and want to be respected. They want to be witnessed and held in mind, to be found attractive and cared for. When unhappiness manifests, as it inevitably does after the romance has ended and disillusionment sets in, it is often confusing to individuals why they should stay or why full commitment is required for creating and sustaining bonds of trust between partners. In order for disillusionment to be transformed into greater intimacy and increased engagement, partners must commit themselves to staying together while facing the challenging process of developing the new psychological and spiritual capacities that are required in a marriage of equals.

This commitment typically takes place in an interpersonal environment in which neither religion nor tradition acts as a larger support for the couple. Dialogue Therapy for Couples, and Real Dialogue as a skill, are designed specifically to meet the needs of today's marriage – a term we use loosely to mean a cohabiting partnership. The skill of Real Dialogue is the core intervention in Dialogue Therapy, and can be learned and used outside of a therapy setting, but within Dialogue Therapy it is optimized by partners being introduced to their underlying emotional dynamics, from their families of origin, and applying those insights at times of emotional threat and stress.

To be more precise about contemporary marriage, commitments based on desire, founded on the ideals of equality and reciprocity, have replaced contracts founded on family traditions or religious identity. Without hierarchy, and with the promise of reciprocity, the new marriage requires enhanced levels of self-awareness and emotional maturity, as well as ongoing and frequent negotiations of conflicts and needs (Coontz, 2005). By contrast, the traditional marriage vow "till death do us part," the foundation of marriage over centuries, was rooted in hierarchy, tradition, and the belief that we should not take our feelings too personally. Partners were in the marriage for the long run to benefit their children and follow family traditions, as well as to conserve or expand family resources (such as a particular trade or business, land ownership, wealth or status within the community). It was as though marriage was viewed as a "corporation" to raise children and conserve resources, and the couple was simply the means to that end (Hochschild, 1989). Typically, individuals stayed in unhappy marriages

DOI: 10.4324/9781003200840-1

"for the sake of the family" and felt proud of themselves for doing so. Seldom now do people feel proud of such a reason for staying.

The contemporary intention to stay "as long as this suits *my* needs" has changed the meaning of marriage. Now we take our feelings very seriously and we make judgments based on them. In place of feeling "good because I am staying for the family," we feel that we have been untrue to ourselves if we stay in a committed relationship in which we feel unseen and unknown. Most individuals in North America would say they are "disempowered" or have "low self-esteem" if they stay in an intimate relationship that no longer meets their emotional needs. We have changed the basis for trust in marriage from long-term impersonal assets (tradition, wealth, family status, and longevity of the contract) to personal emotional attunement and the ability to negotiate and handle conflicts with respect (Coontz, 2005). Our trust in a partner is now predicated, in large part, on whether we feel seen, heard, and known, as well as respected for our point of view, not on some contractual arrangement based on religion, tradition, or longevity of the family. In order to retain our bond in this charged emotional and interpersonal atmosphere, individuals need a clearer understanding of their goals for staying together and the skills required for meeting these goals.

New emotional landscapes and old power struggles

After the initial romance is over, partners inevitably find themselves embroiled in repetitive and deadening power struggles and typically refer to these polarizations as "problems with communication." These struggles are often about differences in styles, opinions, views, or needs, which, if ignored or avoided, can erode feelings of closeness and even make it impossible to work through everyday necessary joint decision-making with respect. Increasingly, such polarizations can seem to transform even the most desirable partner into an "intimate enemy" – someone who knows one well and hurts one precisely (Young-Eisendrath, 1993, 2019). Bids for emotional closeness are then frequently declined by one or both partners after unresolved conflicts and disharmonies make even the most attractive partner seem untrustworthy and intentionally hurtful. At this point, partners may sometimes also turn to pornography or polyamory to try to awaken the vitality of a bond deadened by emotional obstacles to closeness and cooperation (Perel, 2006, 2017). Inevitably these attempts create other anxieties and problems. Ultimately, they backfire and fail because they undermine the security of the primary bond.

Very few people entering into marriage or intimate partnership know much about the requirements for better relational and emotional skills, or the deadening of vitality due to repetitive conflict, or the notion that they must develop as individuals and commit themselves to their relationship. And yet, in order for today's marriage to adapt and survive long enough to become a relationship of equality, partners must learn how to chart a path of responsibility, autonomy, compassion, and witnessing, which must include both truth-telling and the vow of monogamy (even if it is sometimes broken) in order to develop their capacities for staying together. Without these skills and commitment, couples won't thrive. In place of individual psychological and spiritual development that is the promise of a marriage of equals, then, partners will find themselves more thin-skinned, angry, and depressed, or alone in their later years.

The biggest obstacles to emotional attunement and cooperation, occurring in both traditional and contemporary marriages, cluster around "projection" and "projective identification" – forms of unconscious emotional communication and interaction, the labels of which come from psychoanalytic theory. Psychoanalysis (as a theory and a therapy) shows us that much of our emotional communication is unconscious and *habitual*, rooted in early family dynamics that are typically outside our awareness. We will review the concept of *projective identification* in depth in Chapter 3. Here we just introduce it. Please turn to Chapter 3 if you want more details now.

When a characteristic or fault is projected into another person, the projector experiences it as *a part of their perception* of the other person. The projector is shaping a perception, not perceiving another person in reality, but the projector is unconscious of that. The perception simply seems true. In *projective identification*, the receiver of the projection will seem, almost magically, to *produce or exhibit some aspects of* the projected characteristics or behaviors. The receiver of the projection may feel "kidnapped" or triggered in a way that seems to produce what is projected. Further interactions have the uncanny effect, then, of prompting the receiver to "go along" with the projection, which is the "identification" part of "projective identification." Emotional states are evoked and emotional dances are habituated – for example, one partner always seems to the other to be angry, and *angrily* denies the attribution. Couples refer to such rigid dances as "communication problems that we can't seem to overcome" (Johnson, 2008). Both partners become projectors and receivers. Both can seem to identify with a projected quality, attribute, or behavioral pattern expressed through their actions and ways of treating the other person. When a projection seems to be confirmed by the receiver's responses, the sender becomes even more convinced of the "accuracy" of their original "perception" (Klein, 1984; Spillius & O'Shaughnessy, 2012).

This sets up a vicious cycle of blaming another whose behavior apparently confirms the truth of that perception. Typically, this type of projective identification becomes chronic, and can become entrenched, so that partners are unable to handle even the most mundane decision such as, "What color should we paint the kitchen?" Instead of going into a process of inquiry and negotiation, the partners' conversation devolves into accusations ("You always say that!") and defenses ("I was only stating my feelings, don't you want to know my feelings?"). This kind of chronic undermining of cooperative decision-making and ability to talk about differences deadens intimacy and destroys trust, even in the absence of infidelities or outright lying between partners.

Emotional patterns and habits, prominent in our early lives, carry over into our adult lives, both in what is projected into a partner as "ideal" when falling in love, and in what is destructive or negative once disillusionment and power struggles set in. In intimate relationships, projection and identification typically go both ways: each person "directing" a kind of delusional "internal theater" that is at once threatening to their bond *and* to each individual. It is exceptionally difficult for partners to work their way out of these entanglements; the emotions aroused are so powerful and threatening that they provoke further defensiveness, more projective identification, and more retrenchments.

Primacy of intimacy and attunement in the couple

Sadly, in today's couples coming for therapy we find that partners rarely give much priority to their intimacy (sexual or emotional), even though they may both long for it. To make matters worse, partners frequently say that their lack of intimacy is "normal" because the "romance has worn off" and the burdens of a busy life with kids, jobs, and social commitments "don't leave a lot of time for intimacy." Sexual activity may continue in a sort of quid pro quo of each partner's orgasm, but without passion or a feeling of personal connection. Typically, today's partners have spent a lot of time and effort in their search for a "soul mate" or the "right partner." And then, when they feel trapped with an enemy, they assume they have chosen the "wrong person."

That assumption is almost always wrong. Intimacy with an adult partner who is meant to be a friend and an equal requires time and effort and lifelong development. Intimacy is never a simple "done deal." Like a plant or a garden, intimacy is "alive," and it can die if it is not given enough – or the right kind of – attention. Getting into a relationship is planting the seed only. Falling in love is based on mutual idealizing projections, and those projections cannot be sustained after the partnership becomes real, that is, when the quotidian routines of life lose their rosy cast. Instead, the two people must invest in keeping their relationship vital as they become "whole" people, each with weaknesses and limitations, with needs and differences. (The concept of a "whole" person will be discussed in further detail in Chapter 2 in the section titled "Whole self to whole self.")

Today's partners may also have grown up with parents who spent little time together, but had very close emotional bonds with their children, implying that the vitality of the parent-child bond was more compelling and passionate than the partnership between adults. In such a marriage there is an implicit message that adults actually get their emotional needs met through parenting, not through being a couple together.

Chronic unresolved conflicts, projection, and projective identification undermine the health of the marriage and the partners' trust in each other. Then, intimacy is deadened, and partners may feel this circumstance is "normal." The meaning of marriage as an *exclusive* bond between adults in which children are not the center of the stage (as in: "*Our bedroom door is closed*") seems to be an almost foreign idea to many couples coming to therapy. Even when partners fall in love hard, they can become strangers and enemies in a fairly short time and then seek their emotional solace with children or with friends or even pets.

And yet, the bond between parents as partners is the first significant adult relationship that most children *witness* in their young lives. While children have intense relationships *with* their parents, children *witness* the relationship their parents have with each other. Parents become their children's inherent and often unconscious model for how committed partners act and respond to each other. Like Russian nesting dolls, different marriages are nested within each other. Each marriage contains and is contained by the marriages of the partners' individual pasts, as well as those of previous generations. Each marriage also contains the nubbin of future marriages. The unconscious communication and affective meanings in one marriage influence generations of marriages through a set of known and unknown emotional templates that radiate out through the daily lives of children growing up within parental couples (Faimberg, 2005). The parents' marriage is transported into a developing child's relationships with siblings, extended family members, friends, and eventually partners. One of the most important imprints on a child's relationships and bonds is that child's parents' marriage(s).

The internal theater of relational roles and dynamics: Dialogue Therapy

The myriad ways parental couples come together, stay together, and break apart are contained and mirrored in the patterns and templates of an adult's unconscious relational idioms from childhood. Think of our "internal theaters" of relationship as scripted by the idioms or emotional dynamics of the parts played in our early lives by parents, our parents' marriages, siblings, and other important family influencers. These need to be identified and unpacked, in a fundamental way, in the therapeutic environment in order for individuals to perceive how they unknowingly create, through projection and projective identification, specific emotional dynamics that enhance or block intimacy and friendship in their current relationship(s). This discovery process – one of the core aspects of Dialogue Therapy (DT) – involves the exploration of our personal internal theater of desires and fears that exist within the universal constraints and themes (e.g., attachment, separation, loss, or grief) that characterize pair bonds. This discovery process always engenders a deep appreciation of unconscious processes in each and both of the partners, who then feel a new kind of responsibility for their emotional lives.

Dialogue Therapy, in its original form, and as Young-Eisendrath (1984) described it in her book *Hags and Heroes: A Feminist Approach to Jungian Psychotherapy with Couples*, was designed to bring a feminist view into couple therapy and then to allow the therapists to work both with psychodynamics and some aspects of psychodrama with the partners. Young-Eisendrath and her late husband Ed Epstein invented DT, drawing especially on aspects of psychodrama (particularly, "Alter-Ego" and "Role Reversal" techniques) for some of the interventions. They also drew on psychoanalysis, in terms of focusing on projection and projective identification as the primary unconscious obstacles that have to be understood and resolved in order for intimacy to be restored in couples coming for therapy (Young-Eisendrath, 1984).

By creating Dialogue Therapy as a conjoint co-therapy (two therapists with the couple) with a time limit, this method was designed to invite partners, from their first moment in the consulting room, to be responsible for their relationship and their functioning within it, instead of implying that the therapist(s) are responsible to "fix" what is "wrong" with the couple. From its inception, DT was always understood to be more like putting the couple "on stage" and having them "show" who and how they are, than having one partner talk *about* the relationship or to tattle and to "report on" the other partner.

Because Young-Eisendrath is both a psychoanalyst and a feminist (as is Pieniadz), she is and has been profoundly aware of the need for women to be autonomous agents in their own lives and their own individuation. And so Dialogue Therapy came into being with the theme of equality and reciprocity for both partners under the influence of 1980s feminism. The first book she wrote about DT, *Hags and Heroes*, was organized around the thirteenth-century medieval folk story, "The Wedding of Sir Gawain and Dame Ragnelle," in which King Arthur is challenged with the question: "What do women want, above all else?" The answer, which takes a dramatically long time to arrive, is: "They want sovereignty over their own lives, the right to make their own decisions."

Half of *Hags and Heroes* is a Dialogue Therapy training manual for therapists. It was written in the era of Structural Family Therapy and Family Systems Therapy, when family therapists were attempting to "centralize the father" in families in which the "mother dominated," especially in lower income and underserved populations. In the effort to bring fathers back into the family, there was an unintentional silencing of the mothers, often leaving women feeling as though their concerns could not be voiced directly. Dialogue Therapy was designed explicitly to give both partners "equal time" (for example, in the Evaluation and Relational History each partner is empathically interviewed by the therapist to tell their story, while the other observes and may take notes). Also, during Real Dialogue each partner learns specifically to speak for themselves and then to listen mindfully. Each is treated with equal respect in every conflict. Furthermore, the ethos of DT rests on the premise that each partner has equal status. In the 1980s, at the time that *Hags and Heroes* was written, there was a new wave of feminism whereby educated women increasingly assumed leadership roles in the professions, often taking on bread-winning roles in the family while still expected to be responsible for the bulk of parenting and domestic tasks (Hochschild, 1989). Women were also faced with accusations that they "wanted to be men" and that they were moving away from "nurturing." Many women felt angry about shifting conditions that left them unfairly treated in being primary care providers even when they were equal or primary breadwinners. Couples coming to therapy often included an "angry woman" and a "nice man" who has "agreed" to "let" his wife go back to work or school and to "accompany" her into therapy. The repeating scenario of an angry, surly, or depressed woman (the "hag") and a helpful, confused husband (the "hero") who "just didn't get what was going on with his wife, but wanted to help her," was well known in couple therapy and family therapy (Young-Eisendrath, 1984). In profound and eye-opening ways, this presentation of the "hag" and the "hero" was a mirror of the thirteenth-century folk story. Dialogue Therapy therefore highlighted individual sovereignty as the central issue to be addressed through respectful conflict and inquiry between partners over time, as a primary means to their psychological and interpersonal development. Whether in a first marriage or a re-marriage, equality and reciprocity were coming up on the horizon of marriage.

Given these themes of personal sovereignty and equality, Young-Eisendrath and Epstein wanted to create a form of couple therapy that was no longer reliant on a therapist who sits across from two partners (who are themselves typically shoulder to shoulder and not eye-to-eye) and hears their stories, as though the therapist were part of a triangulated situation in which sides might be taken or alliance might be made with one partner or the other. Instead, Dialogue Therapy was devised to be a dramatic set-up in which partners must talk with each other about their reasons for coming to therapy, even at the beginning of the first meeting, rather than *talk to* the therapist. And so the first session of DT always begins with partners facing each other, addressing the following directive: "We (I) would like to hear the two of you talk to each other. We will listen for a while and then we will do something else. Talk about why you are here. Please talk to each other in the ways you typically would, and not to us (me). We will interview each of you later and will get the details." Within this set-up, the couple was always the dramatic scene in which the therapy was unfolding. The therapy would be about the couple, not the therapist's opinion of "what is wrong."

This early, original form of Dialogue Therapy was taught, supervised, and practiced as a conjoint co-therapy with two therapists in the room. The originators did not intend to franchise the practice; they wanted instead to influence the field of couple therapy with their ideas and methods. The originators themselves also enjoyed doing and teaching DT as part of their own development as a couple. The early decades of DT therefore involved small training groups, in which therapists were trained by observing one couple (often a couple in the training group) go through the entire seven co-therapist sessions of DT. After finishing the training, and with *Hags and Heroes* as their training manual, therapists would set out to learn and practice the process on their own while still being supervised by Young-Eisendrath or Epstein. Eventually, of course, they would become full-fledged Dialogue Therapists although there was no official "certification." Because therapists had to train and work together – and typically it was couples who wanted to do that – many people who completed the training were therapists married to each other. Most people who were trained in the early decades of DT loved doing the work and continued doing it throughout their careers until they retired. Dialogue Therapy for Couples was a very small cottage industry in which practitioners engaged in professional conversations with each other, developing their skills over time, and if they were also married to their co-therapist, using DT in their own relationships.

In 1993, Young-Eisendrath published a book about couple relationships, originally titled *You're Not What I Expected: Learning to Love the Opposite Sex*, then re-titled in the paperback edition as *You're Not What I Expected: Love After the Romance Has Ended*. The original title emphasized the difficulty of getting to know the "opposite" sex and the ways that projection and projective identification played a role in entering into a "foreign land" of intimate relating to your "opposite." The book, which was intended to address couples themselves, but was often read and studied by therapists who wanted to learn the method, follows four couples (who are actually collages of couples seen by Young-Eisendrath and Epstein) as they move through the Dialogue Therapy process. The reader sees how partners and relationships change in the course of resolving projective identifications and working through conflicts. These couples epitomize the couples seen in the 1990s in which, compared to the 1980s, women were even more angry, and often very tired, and men even more confused ("I don't know what I am doing here") and despairing ("I don't know what she wants"). One of the couples in *You're Not What I Expected* was based on the couple followed in *Hags and Heroes*, but the others had different concerns. Dramas of step-families, later-life marriages, women breadwinners, open marriages, and multiple divorces had fully come on stage by the 1990s.

Young-Eisendrath and Epstein expanded training in Dialogue Therapy after *You're Not What I Expected* came out, and continued to use *Hags and Heroes* as the training manual. At this point, the issue of needing a co-therapist team in order to do DT was frequently seen as a problem. But the originators held fast to the position that DT is a "container" in which each partner needs to have a therapist. Therefore, the intensity of the method was thought to merit two therapists in the room. The co-therapist model was the only method for doing DT in those days.

In the early 2000s, Young-Eisendrath, a life-long practitioner of Buddhism, began to turn her attention more to Buddhism and the emergence of a dialogue between Buddhism and psychoanalysis. She backed away from supervising and training Dialogue Therapy, but continued to practice with Epstein, who was doing more supervision of the method and practicing it as a solo therapist. In the mid 2000s, Young-Eisendrath and Epstein suffered a tragedy in their personal life: Ed Epstein developed early onset Alzheimer's. From 2004 until Ed's death in 2014, Young-Eisendrath did not practice or teach Dialogue Therapy.

By 2016, Young-Eisendrath had decided that she wanted to bring back Dialogue Therapy and to teach it to a larger professional audience. She felt that contemporary couple therapy failed to address the serious emotional obstacles created by projective identification and the deadening of intimacy that inevitably ensues. As a psychoanalyst and psychologist for individuals, she had had difficulties finding effective referrals for couples among therapists trained in contemporary methods of couple therapy. Too often, it seemed, couples drafted the therapist into their conflicts, and expected the therapist to fix their relationship, and she saw the damage done, then, by the triangulation of the therapist into the couple relationship.

Even worse, she came to understand that many therapists doing couple therapy had little or no special training to work with couples. A major symptom of the failures of couple therapy was the recruitment of the therapist into the relationship by one partner "telling on" the other and making an unconscious alliance with the therapist (an example of projective identification). She saw that couple therapy did not typically produce increased skill or insight in the individual partners. They may have experienced some expansion of knowledge about their history and problems, but that knowledge did not especially help them when projective identification undermined trust during episodes of emotional threat. Too often partners would feel either not helped at all or barely helped by couple therapy. Young-Eisendrath recognized that Dialogue Therapy, with its dramatic short-term focus on projective identification, could be expanded to include the practice of mindfulness through emphasizing the skill of Real Dialogue (RD). She was aware that many people were learning at least a modicum of mindfulness that could be brought to bear on the capacity to contain and simply experience disruptive emotions. She saw that mindfulness could, thus, play a role in resolving the issues of projective identification. Furthermore, she was aware that she would have to adapt DT to a solo therapist model, as we will describe later.

While Young-Eisendrath was in the process of developing the solo model and bringing Dialogue Therapy into a new incarnation, she began to work with Dr. Jean Pieniadz as her co-therapist. Pieniadz and her husband and co-therapist, Joel Shapiro, had both been practicing couple, individual, and family therapy for many years. And they had also been trained by Young-Eisendrath and Epstein in the early format of training, observing live and in real time the full course of a couple going through the process of DT. Working with Pieniadz as co-therapist, and bringing mindfulness practice directly into the method of DT, Young-Eisendrath decided to write another book for couples, taking into account twenty-first century demands on marriage. In 2019, *Love Between Equals: Relationship as a Spiritual Path* came out; it is being read at least as much by therapists as by couples themselves, so we know that therapists are wanting to find out more about DT.

This book closes the circle in bringing into being a new version of Dialogue Therapy and presenting Real Dialogue as an interpersonal mindfulness practice that is used both within DT and beyond clinical settings to address polarization and repetitive conflicts. Since 2016, Young-Eisendrath has developed and carried out full training programs in DT and RD. Pieniadz has been involved in co-teaching some of these programs. Dialogue Therapy training is offered now for licensed mental health professionals. Real Dialogue training is also offered for non-mental health professionals such as life coaches, executive coaches, leaders, human resource managers, mediators, and others. This book is intended to undergird and support the development of skills for those who train and work as Dialogue Therapists and Real Dialogue Specialists.

How does Dialogue Therapy compare to other couple therapies?

As we said earlier, Dialogue Therapy came into being specifically to respond to several flaws or failures in contemporary couple and family therapy. The most important flaw is triangulating of the solo therapist into the couple relationship, as we said earlier, with the therapist consciously or unconsciously taking sides or trying to fix the couple. When partners "report" to the therapist instead of speaking directly to each other, each partner (like a sibling complaining to a parent) knowingly or unknowingly intends to make the other partner "the problem." In fact, sometimes both partners agree that one partner *is* "the problem" – reifying or rigidifying their projective identifications. When the therapist intentionally or unintentionally takes sides or tries to fix either one of the partners or the relationship, then partners may end up being unable to deal with their conflicts without the therapist being present. In our view, the greatest shortcoming of couple therapy is partners becoming dependent on the therapist and thus, instantiating projective identification with the therapist. Couple therapy thus becomes either an ongoing way of life or a revolving door through which the couple enters again and again.

In our view, because couples bring to their therapy a dynamic field of unconscious interactions between partners, there is no need for the therapist to make a special rapport or a positive alliance with either partner. Instead, the therapist is expected *not* to enter that field. Indeed, the Dialogue Therapist "consults on" the interactive field that is already in play between partners. Suffice it to say here that the therapeutic methods, as illustrated in later chapters, are structured in such a way as to keep the focus on either the patterns/dynamics (after the Evaluation is complete) of each partner or on the skills of Real Dialogue that partners are developing. In place of a therapist speaking with a partner *about* the other partner, the Dialogue Therapist is Coaching, Facilitating, Doubling, or Unblocking with one partner. Each treatment session is set up and structured to maximize the distance of the Dialogue Therapist from the "drama" of the couple's internal theater, so that the therapist remains an observer of or expert about the dynamics, even though interpretations of underlying or unconscious processes and motivations may be made either during a session or during the Wrap-Up.

Other contemporary couple therapies take a different approach. The closest to Dialogue Therapy is Harville Hendrix's Imago Therapy (1988/2008), which shares with DT the dramatic set-up for the couple, but differs from DT in significant ways, such as in Imago's use of "homework" and a kind of workshopping of couple's problems. The most significant difference between the two, however, is Imago Therapy's assumption that partners can "work on their relationship" by becoming something like counselors or therapists to each other (*ibid.*). Dialogue Therapy takes the opposite view: partners can never be therapists to each other because of the unconscious entanglements of projective identification that never go away, but *can* be managed through the skills of Real Dialogue. Then, partners become witnesses and remain curious about each other. In other words, in DT, partners learn how to use RD in times of emotional threat and high stress. They learn that each of them lives in a subjective world and that each world is inherently distinct. They learn about each other's vulnerabilities, their emotional habits, and the interactive patterns coming from each partner's early family life. Dialogue Therapy assumes that partners will go on struggling with unconscious entanglements after the therapy ends – but over time that they will become more skillful in dealing with them, and remain wholly engaged witnesses to each other's individuation throughout life together.

Furthermore, in Dialogue Therapy partners become familiar with their differences and learn to respect the space between them. It is that Mindful Gap, the "space between," that allows partners to be attracted to each other, to be playful, and to develop trust (Young-Eisendrath, 2019). This mindful gap is similar to Donald Winnicott's (1971) *play space* or Thomas Ogden's (1993) *dialogical space*. Partners, however, can never be "objective" or even dispassionate about their differences and conflicts. And because of this, they can never be anything like therapists for each other – nor can DT ever replace the role of individual therapy for either partner. So despite some overlapping structures, Dialogue Therapy and Imago Therapy ultimately have different aims and objectives.

Dialogue Therapy has a primary aim of increasing partners' capacities to hold the emotional space open between them and not simply to react, to defend, or to promote themselves. This allows for Witnessing of each other. Dialogue Therapy wants partners to learn how to return freshly to an "I don't know" attitude and a curiosity in which they discover their partner anew.

One of the most popular contemporary couple therapies, Emotion Focused Therapy (EFT), is also quite different from Dialogue Therapy in an important way: EFT targets the couple's attachment needs and styles as the focus of the therapy. EFT assumes that intimate adult relationships are shaped by attachment styles. In couples coming for therapy, attachment styles of avoidance, anxiety, disorganization, or even dismissiveness tend to predominate. A study published in 2010 by Greenberg, Warwar, and Malcolm strongly suggests that if these negative styles or habits can be re-directed towards secure attachment routines, then the couple will recover its optimal emotional, sexual, and interpersonal functioning (pp. 28–43). In a sense, EFT tries to coach the two-person system of the couple to become an optimal attachment system within the limits of the individuals. This is typically done without making each partner fully aware of their history and their own unconscious emotional dynamics. In other words, EFT focuses on the overall dynamics and potentials of the "relationship," and not of the individuals as they interact or become entangled. Of course, EFT wants to analyze the "repetitive cycle" of damaging interaction and then to stop that cycle, but it does so more by imposing an ideal of secure attachment on the

couple than by mapping or charting the projections and projective identifications of each individual.

The EFT therapist plays a major role in convincing partners of "how to fix
their relationship." In 1999, Johnson, Hunsley, Greenberg, and Schindler published research results that demonstrated that a significant number of couples
"feel better" after finishing EFT, but those couples also typically report very
positive feelings about their therapist (pp. 67–79). Something that can be
understood as a "positive transference" to the therapist may be motivating the
good feelings from the therapy. Without the insights and skills to take with
them individually into their future projections, projective identifications, and
polarizations, partners may feel better, but only temporarily, because they are
not really doing better. This is a typical symptom of what in psychoanalysis is
called "transference cure."

Dialogue Therapy aligns with EFT in that adult attachment styles and working
models of attachment are recognized to play a significant role in unconscious and
conscious relational behaviors in equal pair bonds. Nevertheless, DT holds strongly
to the notion that chronic negative projective identification is the primary obstacle
to intimacy (including sexuality), trust, and respectful conflicts in couples who
come to therapy. Without untangling the meanings and habits of these projections,
from each individual into the other, partners will not be able to function as trust-
worthy individuals in their relationship after therapy has ended. Thus, DT departs
from EFT in terms of having the therapist "in charge of" changing the relational
patterns in the couple, the need for a positive transference to the therapist, and the
desire to make the attachment pattern more ideal or secure.

In comparison with the Gottman Method (Gottman, 1994; Gottman &
Schwartz-Gottman 2006, 2015) of behavioral change in couple therapy we
can say that, although partners in Dialogue Therapy are expected to change
their emotional reactivity in the face of repetitive conflicts, DT is not primarily a method aimed at behavioral change. Nor is DT a Cognitive-Behavioral
method. Instead, DT is *experiential*: it places the emphasis on the partners who
will have to differentiate and to incorporate a new perspective on what it
means to retain a mindful gap and respect each other through conflict. Within
this view is an acknowledgement of the irreducible subjective experience of
each partner with their individuality or idiosyncrasy (e.g., Renik, 1999). Consequently, partners become more modest and open-minded without specific
behavioral or cognitive behavioral instruction about these attitudes.

In Dialogue Therapy, partners grasp the importance of the particular skills of
Real Dialogue – Speaking for Yourself, Listening Mindfully, and Remaining
Curious – with an enhanced appreciation of the *complexity* of seeing, hearing, and feeling another person. While Gottman's methods are founded on
his profound insights from his extensive research on couples (e.g., his close
video-taping of research subjects' non-verbal behavior and his tracking of their
emotional activation in conflict), his therapy method arguably does not ask
the couple to build experientially on these insights. Dialogue Therapy draws
on Gottman's research findings to augment our understanding of projective

identification. For example, DT shows partners the threat of their contempt and scorn for each other, and helps them revise it experientially by working through projective identifications. It also bases some of its conception of projective identification on the patterns of unconscious communication depicted in Gottman's research videos.

Whereas Dialogue Therapy differs substantially from Emotion Focused Therapy and the Gottman Method, it shares in some of the assumptions and approaches of the Tavistock method of couple therapy, which also focusses on projective identification. Nevertheless, the Tavistock method does not include the dramatic set-up or the kinds of coaching and facilitating that come from DT's psychodrama background. Within the Tavistock method, the therapist may end up becoming triangulated or giving advice to partners, such as, "You two should spend more time enjoying yourselves together." Though that advice may be founded on a clear understanding of the projective identifications, advice or exhortation does not work without the supportive function of the skills of Real Dialogue.

In Dialogue Therapy, interpretations and facilitation are used to *show* more than to *tell* what is going on between individuals. The partners themselves must be transformed in a palpable way, so they can feel the relief of creating their own *play space* or mindful gap. They come to *experience* the emotional relief in the sessions, not simply be told about it by the therapist. Additionally, when partners finish their treatment program in DT, they make an appointment for one six-month follow-up session (see Chapter 9) in which the Dialogue Therapist(s) watches them go through a Working on a Conflict session, in order to assess and support the skills they have gained. They then graduate, as it were, from Dialogue Therapy. This book will first help you see the arc and the theoretical underpinnings of Dialogue Therapy and Real Dialogue, and then it will describe the sessions and methods in detail.

Bibliography

Coontz, S. (2005). *Marriage, a History: How Love Conquered Marriage*. New York: Penguin.

Faimberg, H. (2005). *The Telescoping of Generations: Listening to the Narcissistic Link between Generations*. London: Routledge.

Gottman, J. (1994). *Why Marriages Succeed or Fail . . . And How You Can Make Yours Last*. New York: Simon & Schuster.

Gottman, J. & Schwartz-Gottman, J. (2006). *10 Lessons to Transform Your Marriage*. New York: Crown Publishers.

Gottman, J. & Schwartz-Gottman, J. (2015). *10 Principles for Doing Effective Couple's Therapy*. New York: W.W. Norton & Company.

Greenberg, L., Warwar, N. & Malcolm, W. (2010). "Emotion-focused couples therapy and the facilitation of forgiveness." *Journal of Marital and Family Therapy*, 36, 28–42.

Hendrix, H. (1998). *Getting the Love You Want: A Guide for Couples (20th Anniversary Edition)*. New York: St. Martin's Griffin.

Hochschild, A. (1989). *The Second Shift: Working Parents and the Revolution at Home*. New York: Viking.

Johnson, S. (2008). *Hold Me Tight: Seven Conversations for a Lifetime of Love*. New York: Little, Brown and Company.

Johnson, S.M., Hunsley, J., Greenberg, L. & Schindler, D. (1999). "Emotionally focused couples therapy: Status and challenges." *Clinical Psychology: Science and Practice*, 6, 67–79. https://doi.org/10.1093/clipsy/6.1.67.

Klein, M. (1984). *Envy and Gratitude and Other Works: 1946–1963*. London: Hogarth Press.

Ogden, T. (1993). *The Matrix of the Mind: Object Relations and the Psychoanalytic Dialogue*. New York: Jason Aronson, Inc.

Perel, E. (2006). *Mating in Captivity: Unlocking Erotic Intelligence*. New York: HarperCollins.

Perel, E. (2017). *The State of Affairs: Rethinking Infidelity*. New York: HarperCollins.

Renik, O. (1993/1999). "Analytic interaction: Conceptualizing technique in light of the analyst's irreducible subjectivity." *Relational Psychoanalysis: The Emergence of a Tradition*. Mitchell, S.A. & Aron, L. (Eds.). New York: Analytic Press.

Spillius, E. & O'Shaughnessy, E. (Eds.). (2013). *Projective Identification: The Fate of a Concept*. New York: Routledge.

Winnicott, D. (1971). *Playing and Reality*. New York: Penguin.

Young-Eisendrath, P. (1984). *Hags and Heroes: A Feminist Approach to Jungian Psychotherapy with Couples*. Toronto: Inner City Books.

Young-Eisendrath, P. (1993). *You're Not What I Expected: Love After the Romance Has Ended*. New York: William Morrow and Company.

Young-Eisendrath, P. (2019). *Love Between Equals: Relationship as a Spiritual Path*. Boulder, CO: Shambala.

2 Increasing trust

Accurate Witnessing versus secure attachment

Contemporary models of relational hygiene and couple therapy typically rest, to some extent, on attachment theory for their rationales and methods. The central notion or theory seems to be that secure attachment is the best foundation for healthy couple relationship between adults (Johnson, 2008). The current notion seems to be that *everyone* would benefit from having more secure bonds. A secure attachment bond is imagined to be a kind of panacea for many ills and the epitome of a lasting trust.

While Dialogue Therapy and Dialogue Therapists embrace the insights of the full range of attachment theory and research, as well as findings on adult attachment styles, forging a more secure attachment bond is not the goal of DT. Dialogue Therapists subscribe to the importance of partners, understanding the models of adult and infant pair bonding, particularly as needed to comprehend separation anxiety and grief, as well as bonding, in their own relationship. Dialogue Therapists may also incorporate self-assessments of adult attachment styles into the Evaluation (e.g., the one that Dr. Diane Poole offers for free online; see: https://dianepooleheller.com/attachment-test/), so that partners can better translate and navigate the differences in their individual attachment styles (Dermendzhiyska, 2020). Even though their attachment styles may change as a result of DT's process, DT does not aim to change the style of either or both partners in a couple.

Instead, Dialogue Therapy bases its major interventions on the theory that individuals become more trusting and intimate as a result of increased differentiation and autonomy, thereby becoming accurate speakers for themselves and witnesses of each other, which may incidentally increase one's sense of security and trust. We make the assumption, based on our clinical experiences with couples, and on research in adult development, that partners and friends trust, respect, and remain interested in each other when they have established an emotional space in which their individuality is accepted and their differing needs can be expressed and negotiated (Schnarch, 1997; Perel, 2006; Young-Eisendrath, 2019). This kind of mindful gap or space allows for authentic relating; it puts an end to, or at least pauses, unbridled desires to control each other's behaviors, feelings, or thoughts. In other words, DT assumes that breaking up chronic projective identifications allows partners to experience the affection, respect,

DOI: 10.4324/9781003200840-2

and desire they genuinely feel for each other. Dialogue Therapy specifically rejects imposing relational *ideals* on partners' behaviors in order to "make the relationship more secure or loving."

However, Dialogue Therapists help partners to understand the general meanings of *attachment bond, separation anxiety,* and *grief* in adult pair bonding. For example, when partners make "separation threats" (threatening to leave or abandon the other) as a means of trying to convince or persuade the other person of the seriousness of some situation, they learn in Dialogue Therapy that such threats *increase* anxiety, sometimes fostering rage or protest. Thus, separation threats undermine partners' ability to handle the problem-solving or decision-making at hand. After clients understand what separation anxiety is, they can more readily agree that separation threats are damaging.

In place of valorizing secure attachment, Dialogue Therapy emphasizes the function of Witnessing (also called *objective empathy*), which requires stepping outside one's own subjectivity without necessarily endorsing or agreeing to the other person's reality, and learning the three skills of Real Dialogue: Speaking for Yourself, Listening Mindfully, and Remaining Curious. These are needed to help partners restore and maintain trust, respect, and intimacy between them.

While a secure attachment bond conveys *feelings* of trust (e.g., comfort and ease), it does not necessarily enhance or develop a person's ability to see, hear, and feel the other person accurately – to become an accurate witness – or to speak for oneself. The attitudes or behaviors associated with secure attachment (e.g., feeling both confident and vulnerable within the attachment bond) are sometimes recommended or exhorted by couple therapists in an attempt to increase trust or warmth. But those exhortations may instead unintentionally lead to increased enmeshment and projective identification if one person *commands* the other (equal partner) to engage in certain behaviors in order "to increase our love" or "to be loving." Also, an adult attachment bond can be undermined rapidly and even permanently in a single heated conflict in which one or both people humiliates the other or repeatedly threatens separation, even if no one becomes violent or otherwise destructive. Making or intending a secure attachment with another person *does not automatically enhance our skills* in Witnessing that person accurately, as any securely attached parent knows when their children become teenagers and then adults.

Different capacities and skills are needed for Witnessing than for secure attachment. Accurate Witnessing and respect for another's limitations and differences go beyond emotional attunement and sometimes beyond emotional intelligence. Witnessing is an interactive skill that is rooted in mindfulness and curiosity, as well as compassion for both parties.

Witnessing and Real Dialogue depend on these three things: (1) emotional and psychological differentiation; (2) capacity for mindfulness (concentration plus equanimity); and (3) a multifaceted ability to contain and cognize one's own subjectivity. In order to grow and develop the ability to see, hear, and feel another person who seems to be emotionally threatening or demanding a particular outcome (e.g., "I want to make you happy!") we all need specific skills and capacities. But, negative projective identification blocks such capacities and then affects the ways that partners see each other in terms of "being loved."

If couple therapists do not recognize projective identification and the enmeshment and confusion it brings into relationship, then partners may be thrown into despair or argument about whether the other person really "loves" them. Whether projective identification is idealizing, as in falling in love, or devaluing and devitalizing as in disillusionment and polarization, it affects partners' problem-solving, decision-making, grieving, and gratitude (even when it's idealizing) in ways that are troubling to the sense of "being loved" and "met" by the other. For example, if the bond or the partner is idealized, then one or both partners may believe that the other person should "be able to know without asking or saying" exactly what needs to be done to meet one's needs. There may also be a belief that by simply voicing one's needs (e.g., "I need some help here"), they should be met if one is "truly loved." Under these conditions, partners will try to manage or control each other so their "love" is not disproven. On the other hand, if the bond is devalued or devitalized (because of a deadening projective identification), then partners may not even voice their needs because they feel unseen and unknown. And so, projective identification intersects with the ways that therapists and clients cognize and feel about attachment bonds and the nature of love or getting needs met. Moreover, projective identification is a relational variable that is independent of any individual's attachment style (Fonagy, Gyorgy, Jurist & Target, 2004).

And yet, once the obstacle of projective identification is sufficiently diminished, then differences between partners can be witnessed, and even differences in attachment styles can be known and discussed, allowing partners to accept the different styles of meeting needs that exist between them as individuals. But if secure attachment and an idealized love are valorized by a couple therapist, then the therapist and partners will tend to confuse meeting needs with love. And the couple bond may be constantly threatened if needs are not met as each partner desires.

The expanse between

The poet Rainer Maria Rilke (1975) famously wrote:

> Once the realization is accepted that even between the closest people infinite distances exist, a marvelous living side by side can grow up for them, if they succeed in loving the expanse between them.

Dialogue Therapy emphasizes partners' abilities to witness the emotional space between them without closing down that space – e.g., with the urge to control or manage the other person's perceptions or actions to get wished-for outcomes or to defend against fears. We find that when individuals feel seen, heard, and known by each other, then partners are able to take up the tasks of intimacy-building, problem-solving, respectful conflict, and trust repair. This also means that partners can affirm their individuality, as well as tolerate annoying differences and limitations. The reciprocal experience of seeing, hearing, and feeling in a partnership brings tremendous emotional relief and increases trust at every level of relating (Young-Eisendrath, 2019). By engaging in activities and skills that bring about these outcomes, partners will spontaneously discover that the skills are self-rewarding and self-organizing. Once individuals have a fundamental acceptance of each other's habits and limitations (rather than taking them "personally"), then all sorts of other capacities unfold as needed, leading to ongoing growth in emotional intelligence, psychological maturity, intimacy, ease, and even spiritual meaning. It is our contention that partners and other relational equals (e.g., adult children and parents) must learn to communicate subjectively and respectfully about their conflicts in order to establish a harmony that continues through the years. Any harmony that is imposed as "rules for love," or any other model advancing a picture of "the ideal relationship," can easily become a potential threat if one person demands fulfillment of the ideals over true love for the other individual as they are.

For example, "nonviolent communication" (Rosenberg, 2015), when it is a demand on speakers for negotiating needs, tends to reinforce passive aggression when individuals do not get their emotional needs met, and then as a consequence do not feel free to speak authentically from a subjective point of view, but instead feel ashamed of their aggression (Siegel, 1999, pp. 65–85). The emphasis on Speaking for Yourself and Listening Mindfully in Real Dialogue offers a fresh approach to establishing harmony that comes from the foundational ability to trust self and other to work through conflicts without restricting the subjective validity of either individual.

The couple's theater: two people in a relationship

From beginning to end, Dialogue Therapy provides a therapeutic environment that is like an improvisational theater. Each new couple discovers their own differentiated interactions with each other, alongside the therapists' support, but not through the therapists' ideals being imposed on them. Not only do partners face each other in most of the sessions, but Dialogue Therapists function not so much as "interpreters" or "judges" of the relationship, but more as facilitators, coaches, referees, and "Alter-Egos" for individual partners (more on this later). The role of Dialogue Therapists, throughout the process of treatment, is to make themselves less and less necessary to the actual communication of the partners. At the start, therapists are active and involved in lengthier interventions, but they become *less* active as the process moves toward its end.

Helping couples understand and appreciate differentiation means that Dialogue Therapists endorse the role of autonomy and personal responsibility as keys to healthy functioning in partners or other equal dyads. Dialogue Therapy sharpens partners' capacities to experience both themselves and the other as "subjectivities" or as "separate worlds of subjective experience" that cannot be boiled down to a single formula. The primary means of doing this is having partners actively involved in working through their conflicts using Real Dialogue while repeatedly inviting them to develop empathy in becoming witnesses – first through the processes of the Evaluation and then, finally, through the experience of Role Reversal. At no point along the way do Dialogue Therapists interpret "the relationship" as secure, insecure, anxious, avoidant, or the like. Instead, Dialogue Therapists focus their interventions and facilitation on two individuals – who may have quite different attachment and personality styles – relating to each other, consciously and unconsciously.

Mindful gap

The emotional expanse between partners is called a *mindful gap* in the language of Dialogue Therapy. This idea, as mentioned earlier, originates with Winnicott's (1957/1992) theory of *play space* and Ogden's (1993) notion of *dialogical space*. These are interpersonal emotional spaces in which people feel free to relate and to be themselves, accompanied by humor and creativity or grief and vulnerability. These psychoanalytic concepts of emotional space point to the necessity of engaging and accepting the differences between our own and another's subjectivity, in order to feel close or to have a relationship. If instead we assume that we see, hear, and feel things "exactly like" someone else does, then we have no curiosity about their experience, and we can make quick and sometimes dangerously inaccurate attributions about their intentions or motives (Perel, 2006). Collapsing the emotional space between partners provokes self-protection and self-defense in both people, especially at times of threat when one person feels swept up into or hostile about the other's needs, desires, or control. In fact, the main reason why today's couples come to therapy, or why other kinds of pairs or partnerships seek facilitation for "difficult conversations," is that each individual feels there is "no space to be myself," that "I can't solve problems with this person because we keep getting hijacked into the same repetitive conversations." This is not, in fact, a "communication problem." It is a problem of projective identification or unconscious affective communication that goes far beyond words (Caper, 2020).

Without a gap or a space between us, we are either fused and enmeshed (with a demand to "see it, hear it, or feel it" just "as I say you should") or emotionally estranged (as in the complaint, "You never understand what I try to tell you, no matter what I say") because there is a refusal to admit any differences. Individuals then feel that if they do not "match" each other, something is either bad, wrong, or failing – an experience and a label most anyone in a couple wants to avoid. Such avoidance can lead to further misunderstanding, as well as a devitalizing experience of the relationship, with little room for play, uses of metaphor, humor, sexual relating, or any affective colorations that lend to their dynamism the potential for novelty and surprise.

Learning how to maintain a mindful gap in one's relationship provides a basis for optimal experiences of autonomy, relationality, and responsibility in adult life. Adults who are able to work within the constraints of their own subjectivity will naturally come to recognize that they can witness a partner only when they *are able to tolerate their own experiences* and hold them in such a way as to make room for another.

Love as psychological and spiritual development

Holding open a mindful gap and inquiring into the emotional habits of oneself and another provide a path for ongoing individuation and development in adult life. Two people can then actualize the individuation process with each other, not through acting as each other's therapist, but by being accurate witnesses, remaining curious, and appreciating each other's subjectivities for their different flavors and meanings. In this way, both people are compelled to experience self and other fully and clearly, as whole selves, while accepting the limitations of each person and of the relationship. As a result, instead of simply threatening the relationship or making unwieldy demands via unconscious communications and projections, partners are invited into greater insights and compassion, as they use the skills of Real Dialogue over the decades, and explore their experiences at each new stage of an ongoing life together. Is it possible for each partner to value the other as an equal, not more or less, in developing new insights and capacities? Dialogue Therapy says *yes*. Becoming an accurate witness and maintaining a mindful gap – with a partner, a friend, a parent, or a grown child – requires the development of, and ongoing access to, three aspects of mindfulness: concentration, equanimity, and vulnerability (i.e., surrendering one's need to control the other).

In an essential way, loving our equal demands that we pay *close attention* – concentrating on their being – as we know them over time. Through facilitating, demonstrating, and coaching, Dialogue Therapy provides regular opportunities for partners to practice mindfulness skills within and outside of sessions. Giving up one's desire to control or change the other is a sacrifice that becomes a kind of "spiritual" practice of acceptance, founded on one's ability to tolerate and contain one's own emotional reactivity.

When it comes to being loved – not simply wanted or desired – we are all sensitive to how we are seen or felt: no one wants to be emotionally used, managed, ignored, or controlled. Through Dialogue Therapy, partners learn how to bear, and bare, their vulnerability and to show the particularity of their own needs, whether or not those needs can be met. Baring our hearts with their particularities can lead to feeling painfully wounded if the listener distorts, misunderstands, or ignores us, *especially if that person is our partner*. At these times, engaging in dialogue and making room for a mindful gap is the practice of choice. In DT, couples also learn that Real Dialogue might not always be possible or might need to be delayed, and at those times individuals must be able to address their own needs and wants, and to contain their emotional reactivity until partners can speak together using their Real Dialogue skills.

In all these ways, working within a mindful gap means working with one's own subjective experience and making a space in which to see, hear, and feel another's subjectivity. *Experiencing* feelings, thoughts, and body sensations is not the same thing as *expressing* them. The mindful gap between partners means that we can *experience* our own subjective world without necessarily having to *express* it. In Dialogue Therapy, partners learn that there are three nonexclusive options regarding feelings and thoughts: express, suppress, or *experience*. Learning this discernment of our emotions and feelings leads to ongoing psychological development.

Although partners always come to Dialogue Therapy with chronic and repetitive power struggles that are entangled in painful projections and enmeshments, they will leave with much more than the sorting-out of these issues. They will leave with the skills and insights to inquire into themselves and their relationship, repeatedly after the therapy is over, in order to take back and examine harmful and hurtful projections. They will also leave with a new interest in their childhood wounds and traumas as these open doors to greater self-understanding, compassion, and kindness. Painful distortions in how partners see each other will not, however, simply disappear. The themes of these distortions will become familiar so that individuals can learn to respond to emotional imprints from the past with increased care and comfort in themselves and their relationship. This increases the space in which two people can regard each other as whole self to whole self over time.

Whole self to whole self

As adults we have the possibility of developing psychological capacities that move beyond secure attachment, and even emotional intelligence, through our relationships with our partners, grown children, siblings, and friends. When we experience ourselves as a "whole self" we are embodying our own authentic being with all of its complexities, strengths, habits, and weaknesses. We are no longer ashamed or afraid of our limitations because we recognize them as part and parcel of a human self. We experience, and may even express, both the creativity and the vulnerability of our own nature. When someone who knows us well can become an ongoing witness to this whole self, we feel more alive and engaged with our own being. When we can do this for another, we feel a tremendous relief in being able to love another person without wanting to change a hair on their head!

This kind of developmental achievement – loving the whole human self as we find it – is the seed that Dialogue Therapy hopes to plant in partners. We do this through the Evaluation (as each partner observes the other's interview), and then through the comprehensive process of Coaching, Facilitating, Doubling, and Unblocking in Real Dialogue. And finally, we cap the process off with the Role Reversal interview that assesses, at the end of DT, both partners' empathy and Witnessing capacities. The entire sequence of DT's sessions was designed so that partners could engage with their ongoing autonomy, vulnerability, and deepened meaning in each other's lives.

Autonomy

The idea of autonomy – literally *self-governance* – is very much a Western psychological concept. And yet it is an important component to any adult life. It includes the right to pursue happiness, to make decisions, to speak for ourselves, to make choices, and even to take risks, within the strictures of our laws. These are aspects of adulthood that most of us cherish and that we must surrender if we fall ill in a way whereby we can no longer take care of ourselves. When it comes to love between equals, the role of autonomy is important and respect for it is a priority. To commit to a partner, to move in together, to share finances, to plan a household life, to raise children, is a matter of continuous negotiation so that each person's autonomy is respected. Necessarily, that means that partners' differing needs and desires will not be met perfectly, but must be understood and witnessed, and then worked with until each person feels "good enough" about agreed-upon methods and strategies that are embraced.

Real Dialogue within the course of Dialogue Therapy repeatedly emphasizes that each person is an adult and that neither one can take "command" or "control" of the other or claim to be simply more injured or victimized than the other. Neither partner is allowed to occupy the "moral high ground" of being "justified" in attacking the other person. Even when injuries are real and painful, each partner needs to investigate and ameliorate their own role in the injuries. In fact, at every step of the way in the DT process, therapists make a concerted effort to reinterpret and redirect attempts to scapegoat or to blame a partner. Neither adult can "make" the other do something without that other's consent. This is part of being in an adult relationship.

However, Dialogue Therapy is contraindicated when individuals have certain kinds of impulsive behaviors such as active untreated addictions to drugs and alcohol, untreated suicidal or homicidal impulses or plans, active untreated domestic violence, or a prevalence in one or both people of a psychotic disorder. (Chapter 5 offers more information about contraindications for DT). Dialogue Therapy is suitable only when its constraints and methods are a reasonable match to partners' situations and capacities.

It is clear to Dialogue Therapists that close personal relationships – whether in marriage, co-habitation, friendship, or parenting – move from idealization and fantasy to disillusionment and reality. This process means that individuals fall into negative views of each other and have perceptions of the other person as being "at fault" for what is painful and disappointing. In the process of Dialogue Therapy, partners are encouraged to see more clearly into the bigger picture of their own life circumstances – in terms of the emotional themes, traumas, and losses in childhood – and the experience of feelings and emotions that motivate (often unconsciously) actions and language. Dialogue Therapists repeatedly return to the idea that "You have a choice" when speaking with partners, to emphasize that each of us has a choice in the ways we see, hear, and feel our experiences: we can take a step back from our initial reactivity and get a bigger view, as well as contain or restrain our impulse to accuse, blame, or leave the conversation. Partners and other dyads have the freedom to stay or leave, even to stay or leave the DT process. No one is "making" anyone choose, stay, or feel in any particular way. This is what autonomy means. We have subjective freedom to work with our own minds, attitudes, and experiences. We also have the ability to forgive ourselves and others for mistakes and other limitations.

To become an accurate Witness and maintain a mindful gap, each client recognizes that a partner, friend, or grown child cannot, does not, and will not want exactly the same things as oneself. While we are always free to leave or separate, we will also experience the rupture of leaving as grief and loss. Once we have entered into an attachment bond, there is no absolute freedom. We have to accept the constraints of retaining a relationship or choosing the grief of separating. These choices make our love more poignant. We do not "have to" submit to the "common good" as it might seem in a "till-death-do-us-part" style of marriage; but in order to grow and develop with another person, we must willingly choose to stay again and again, and to learn again and again, how to mind the gap of our differing subjectivities. In Dialogue Therapy, partners learn to accept both their own and the other's limitations and to express vulnerabilities until they are *witnessed*, even if their needs cannot be met by the other person. In doing all this, partners learn how to feel their own feelings, to express them as they choose, and to take their hurts less personally. More and more, they will learn what it means to be a Witness to whole self and whole other.

By surrendering the desire to control or manage the other person, partners in Dialogue Therapy come to understand what it means to allow another person to be a whole self. Truly surrendering control of the beloved can be confusing for many. Mothers, especially, may have developed a sincere belief that controlling another's habits or desires is "helpful" or even "life-saving." When young children are at home, parents need to control and manage their children's emotional and physical needs in order to keep them safe and thriving. But after the age of seventeen or so, children should be able to become increasingly more autonomous by asking for help or guidance while parents generally and incrementally surrender control of their well-being and safety, except when asked. Of course, we all fall prey to the idea that we can help another not to go down the "wrong path," as it were, when that help is clearly not wanted.

But in DT, partners learn that they must first ask: "Do you want some feedback?" or "Would you like some help with that?" Partners may then find that the other person may decline and that that decline needs to be accepted. The "right size" gap between any two adults needs to be large enough for both people to feel autonomous and be able to consult their own subjectivity, but not so large that individuals feel isolated and emotionally out of contact. Sometimes, people might even need to live on different coasts in order to feel the "right-sized" mindful gap within their partnership!

Vulnerability, sexuality, and intimacy

As partners learn about their autonomy and their right to choose again and again, as well as the skills and capacities to develop together as accurate Witnesses, both will start trusting more in their relationship, expressing their feelings, and then their vulnerability can grow. Trust grows because each individual knows that their own differences and styles will not undermine the bond between them. Vulnerability grows because each person feels the emotional exposure of having to ask for what they need and to know something about their own (and the other person's) feelings, especially their wounds and hurts and discouragements. Vulnerability comes into play as partners want to be cared about or supported. These desires, mostly, have to be put into words. They have to be expressed in a way that is not blaming or attacking. The partner, however, might not be equipped to respond as the speaker hopes or the partner may not want to respond because of needs or desires of their own. Alternatively, the partner might try to respond and fail, or sometimes fail and sometimes not. All of these experiences can increase one's sense of vulnerability. But in the Dialogue Therapy process, partners come to tolerate and learn from their vulnerability, and begin to see it as necessary for being in a loving partnership.

Another reason why two people in a dyad can experience and embrace their own weaknesses and limitations is that they have moved away from the ideal that a couple or pair (e.g., siblings or a child-parent relationship, etc.) must function in a *certain* way; that the dyad must, for example, always be in harmony, or eliminate differences, or that we must "always do our best." People may impose these kinds of ideals and use them for "cheerleading," or seemingly inspiring kindness, while also experiencing them as slightly, or grossly, oppressive.

Expression, response, and failure necessarily cycle through true love, with no end. They also cycle through Real Dialogue. We can never know another person perfectly, because, we never know ourselves perfectly. And we all change with circumstances, time, and age. Needs change and desires change. This is why the ongoing expression of needs and desires can be experienced as poignant or touching. As partners become better Witnesses in Dialogue Therapy, they typically feel a tremendous relief in being able to talk about their issues without a pressure to solve, compromise, or meet the other's needs. There is a relief in minding the gap and also in Witnessing the vulnerability in self or other when needs cannot be met. This kind of Witnessing increases intimacy, as you will later see in the case material (e.g., Chapter 8). Witnessing and differentiation break through the pressures of projective identification, leaving both partners feeling enlivened, even when they cannot become what is wanted by the other person.

Through the course of Dialogue Therapy, partners are encouraged to become familiar with limitations in each other. This assists both people in feeling their dependency needs more strongly and recognizing how dependency changes over time − from perhaps passionate needs early in the relationship, to later needs for support, as well as needs for friendship and co-parenting, and still later, to needs for help with aging, illness, and the loss of loved ones. The desire to be Witnessed and recognized is ever-present. People want to be seen, heard, and felt as individuals, even if others cannot do or say exactly what the person is seeking (Benjamin, 2018).

The mindful gap makes room for the acceptance of successes, ambitions, limitations, and imperfections in both adults. This acceptance gives new space for sexual desires and styles. Dialogue Therapists assume that sexuality is *part of relating*, not something separate. We assume that a well-functioning couple will be able to have an engaged and engaging dialogue about what they want sexually together. If a couple is merged or enmeshed through projective identification, then each person may feel controlled by the other: e.g., one person might feel "obliged" to have sex while the other person might feel "blamed" or "scolded" for "having too many needs."

Both or either might feel ashamed of their own desires, or guilty for not meeting the other's. When partners are merged, they try to guess at and accommodate each other's needs without getting a full picture of what the other person needs or wants, or what the other finds exciting or feels upset about. For instance, a partner might use pornography for masturbation in order not to "bother" the other person, despite never having checked in with that other person. Projective identification leaves partners feeling like they must suppress, dampen, or deny what is taking place within or between them, as regards their sexual and intimate needs. This is because they cannot seem to tolerate the feelings aroused by the sense of not fulfilling their own or their partner's needs (Young-Eisendrath, 2019).

Real Dialogue skills and insights gleaned from accurate Witnessing reduce the self-conscious feelings of shame and guilt that often undermine partners' desires to be close. Those feelings typically keep people focused on themselves, not on their relationship, and on the partner.

In the course of Dialogue Therapy, partners begin to understand that sex and intimacy are matters of practical pleasures and desires, not personal referendums on how much they are "wanted" or whether they are attractive or desirable. They begin to speak about orgasm and pleasure in terms of what feels good and how they enjoy this or that. Together, then, partners can find creative ways to meet some or most of each other's needs (Perel, 2006, 2017). Indeed, intimate encounters, like conversations, are a way to learn about how someone else has pleasure and release. Getting to sexual pleasure for both people is often one goal of Real Dialogue, and if an orgasm is not possible (e.g., because of health limitations), then at least getting to pleasure for both is aspirational. There are many ways for adults to achieve sexual pleasure and excitement together. Partners can talk about this in a way that shows respect for their differences, while also showing interest in finding creative ways to access or attain what is possible between them. At different periods of the lifecycle, different kinds of vulnerability and sexual activity are highlighted for any individual. These aspects of being an adult change, just like everything else in life.

Purpose and meaning in individual lives

With regard to nourishing deep meaning and purpose in our lives, the couple (and other relationships) can take center stage in supporting that development, provided both people are able to maintain a mindful space in which each individual can remain interested in the other's world. Near the end of Dialogue Therapy, partners engage in what is called a Role Reversal interview in which each partner of the dyad is interviewed as though they were the other person. By this point in the process, both partners have had to demonstrate their ability to use their Real Dialogue skills and to embrace the insights from the Evaluation about the underlying emotional limitations and liabilities of self and other. In the Role Reversal, each person has an opportunity to take a deep dive into the world of the other.

Dialogue Therapists conduct this Role Reversal interview in a way that touches on each person's purpose or meaning in life, and how that is supported or unsupported by their partner, so that each can Witness being heard and felt by the other. Typically, clients find this activity of Role Reversal both refreshing and surprising, as it reinforces their desire to relate more intimately; they feel seen, heard, and encouraged to speak about what might be left out or inaccurate. Over time, a well-functioning dyad should be able to offer support for each other's individuation process. By this, we mean showing both interest in and knowledge of the creative, spiritual, socio-political, or work developments of the other person. Real Dialogue on these topics always means leaving management and control in the other person's hands.

Through Role Reversal, and by practicing Real Dialogue in therapy and at home, clients learn how to offer suggestions or help in ways that are welcomed by the other. For example, if there are big differences that need to be negotiated in order for one person to go back to school or change jobs, then the two need to use RD to slow down the process of problem-solving until each person clearly understands the other's views and concerns. They will find that they cannot rush toward closure on any big topic in the arena of purpose and meaning in each other's lives.

When two people have significant differences, they need to be careful not to assume that they share assumptions or desires. The key to mutual discovery and happiness in dialogue about the bigger meanings and purposes in each other's lives is to be able to Witness – to hear accurately and to accept – the other's sense of purpose and meaning. There also needs to be curiosity in hearing about the details, as well as compassion in noticing the suffering and disappointments.

What Real Dialogue repeatedly shows us is that partners do not need to resolve their differences, compromise, or share common ground, but only need to create the emotional space in which each person can speak for oneself, listen mindfully, and check out the accuracy of what has been heard and understood. Under those conditions, individuals can find a way to solve the practical problems between them. But if either feels that one must buckle under the other's needs, or that the other is dismissive or uninterested in their heart's most important meanings, then trust evaporates. Trusting a relationship to go on means that both people trust they can be themselves fully and wholly – or, put differently, that they don't need to sacrifice the core of their individuality in order to embrace or enjoy the relationship.

Healthy bodies, desires, finances, living situations, social networks: these are just some of the things that change throughout years and decades for couples. Relating whole self to whole self, every step of the way, through the changing landscapes of life and purpose, means that partners and friends can work with their circumstances as they age, without threatening their bond. Knowing you will be accepted as you change within the bigger picture of your life also enhances the mystery about *what is unfolding within each individual as time passes.* The two people are able to speak for themselves and their own subjectivity with a freedom and authenticity, because they know that the other person will be interested in, curious about what is happening. As two people evolve in such a way, they find their love to be both familiar and mysterious, both comforting and exciting, both pleasurable and challenging.

Constraints and limitations of individuals

In the course of Dialogue Therapy, not everyone is equal in being able to use the Real Dialogue skills and to tolerate childhood and other traumas that are re-wounded in the current relationship. Relating whole self to whole self sometimes means that one person (who, for example, has physical disease or psychological symptoms) has to accept and tolerate a lack of Witnessing from the other because that other (who might also have limiting conditions) does not have the emotional bandwidth or freedom to listen mindfully. If that becomes the case, then Dialogue Therapists will talk with the clients about strategies that allow for the relational bond to be strengthened as much as possible given these particular forms of differentiation of the two individuals. Psychological defenses and physical impairments (e.g., a fatal illness) can limit another's ability to see, hear, and feel someone else's subjectivity accurately and, of course, those kinds of limitations might also interfere with a person's ability to listen mindfully during conflict.

Thus, Dialogue Therapists recognize that people are not equal in their ability to use the skills of dialogue. Nor is anyone able to perfect these skills in all circumstances. But when these skills fail, the clients should know generally what to do in order to maintain differentiation and prevent chronic projective identification from dominating. Through the entire course of Dialogue Therapy, the therapists emphasize themes of personal responsibility in order for partners to work within themselves to become better Witnesses. We know that accurate Witnessing depends on mindfulness in any given moment. Keeping emotional threat levels as low as possible and working realistically with a particular couple's ability to use the skills of Real Dialogue is not only a goal, but also the path of successful Dialogue Therapy.

Bibliography

Benjamin, J. (2018). *Beyond Doer and Done To: Recognition Theory, Intersubjectivity, and the Third.* London: Routledge.

Caper, R. (2020). *Bion and Thoughts Too Deep for Words: Psychoanalysis, Suggestion, and the Language of the Unconscious*. New York: Routledge.

Dermendzhiyska, E. (2020, January 10). "How you attach to people may explain a lot about your inner life." *The Guardian*. Retrieved from www.theguardian.com/science/2020/jan/10/psychotherapy-childhood-mental-health.

Fonagy, P., Gyorgy, G., Jurist, E. & Target, M. (2004). *Affect Regulation, Mentalization, and the Development of the Self*. New York: Other Press.

Johnson, S. (2008). *Hold Me Tight: Seven Conversations for a Lifetime of Love*. New York: Little, Brown and Company.

Ogden, T. (1993). *The Matrix of the Mind: Object Relations and the Psychoanalytic Dialogue*. New York: Jason Aronson, Inc.

Perel, E. (2006). *Mating in Captivity: Unlocking Erotic Intelligence*. New York: HarperCollins.

Perel, E. (2017). *The State of Affairs: Rethinking Infidelity*. New York: Harper.

Rilke, R.M. (1975). *Rilke on Love and Other Difficulties* (Mood, J., Trans.). New York: W.W. Norton & Company, Inc.

Rosenberg, M.B. (2015). *Nonviolent Communication: A Language of Life*. Encinitas, CA: Puddle Dancer Press.

Schnarch, D. (1997). *Passionate Marriage: Love, Sex, and Intimacy in Emotionally Committed Relationships*. New York: W.W. Norton & Company.

Siegel, J.P. (1999). "Destructive conflict in nonviolent couples." *Journal of Emotional Abuse*, 1(3), 65–85. https://doi.org/10.1300/J135v01n03_04.

Winnicott, D. (1992). *The Child, the Family, and the Outside World*. New York: Perseus Publishing.

Young-Eisendrath, P. (2019). *Love Between Equals: Relationship as a Spiritual Path*. Boulder, CO: Shambala.

3   Projective identification as unconscious interaction

Whether or not you are familiar with the term *projective identification*, you have been affected by the experience of projective identification. Projective identification is not abstract. It is a direct experience that all of us have. It refers to interactions with others in which you seem to be captured or kidnapped by their emotions or emotional meanings, and then carried into a kind of "script" or "tape" in a way that you had not intended. Often, you will notice this kind of unconscious communication in individual therapy with someone who "rocks your boat" – for example, you forget something obvious about the person just after they tell you how sensitive they are about such forgetting, you can't recall their name at the end of a difficult session, or you say something to them that is overly personal that you did not intend to say.

Projective identification happens outside of therapy, too, of course. It happens when we are interacting with our partner or other family members (e.g., parents, siblings, children), or with friends and co-workers.

Projective identification is a psychological process that includes or consists of any and all of the following: a type of defense, a mode of communication, a form of relating to another person emotionally, and an opening to psychological change (Ogden, 1991). Across these modes, projective identification may be a communication of something *with* someone; an expelling or externalizing of something *into* someone; an attempted control *of* someone; or an emotional assault *on* someone (Caper, 2000). Within the drama of projective identification many kinds of interactions may be taking place, used for different purposes, all of which may be subconscious, partly conscious, or wholly unconscious.

For example, in Dialogue Therapy, when the couple enters the room and sits down, the therapists say something along these lines: "I'd like to hear the two of you talk with each other. I'd like to hear you talk about your reasons for being here. You don't need to worry about giving me the background, because each of you will be interviewed for that. Just talk together now about why you are here and what you hope to get from this experience." At least eighty percent of the time, one person says "Why don't you begin?" or "Do you want to begin?" Of course, that person *has already begun*! And if the statement seems insistent that the *other* person speak first, then the speaker is taking control of the interaction, saying that the other person *should* speak first. The recipient of the message then

DOI: 10.4324/9781003200840-3

feels a pressure to comply and typically does begin to speak. This is a quick and apparently simple moment of one type of projective identification in which one person embodies the *puppeteer* and the other becomes the *puppet* – the first person is taking *control of* the second.

A brief history of the term

In 1946, the British psychoanalyst Melanie Klein described in her paper, "Notes on Some Schizoid Mechanisms," a phenomenon that she had seen in young children with whom she was working in psychoanalysis. It consisted of the children describing unconscious fantasies of expelling unbearable parts of their minds into others and taking parts of others' minds into their own – introjection. This balance of projection and introjection Klein eventually called "projective identification" (Klein, 1946/1984). She observed that this function both resulted from and supported the fantasy that one's mind was not separate or discrete from other minds, which we can imagine as a kind of preverbal synchronizing of minds through influence and contact in both imagining and projecting. Projective identification, Klein discovered, eventually evolves into the child's attempts to manage experiences in order to communicate with others on whom the child depends (*ibid.*). Of course, infants and young children are very complex and extremely helpless organisms and are faced with a barrage of complicated and frightening stimuli that need to be organized and shaped through interactions.

Through projective identification with caregivers, the child gradually develops the ability to keep painful, dangerous, and frightening experiences sorted separately from comforting, soothing, and calming ones (*ibid.*). This kind of "splitting" of the "bad" from the "good," pain from pleasure, is an early development of a psychological defense to project the "bad things" or painful experiences "outside" oneself, and to take and hold the "good" ones "inside."

Psychological stability takes time to form in infancy. The mothering one(s) play an important role in that they have to be empathic in accurately picking up emotional signals from the infant and helping the infant sort out the meanings. As Winnicott (1956) said, "[o]nly if the mother is sensitized in a way . . . can she feel herself into the infant's place, and so meet the infant's needs" (p. 302).

The infant develops projective identification as a mode of communication that serves primarily defensive and developmental functions. Projective identification is the means by which the infant gets the mother(s) to feel what the infant is feeling, or, alternatively, cannot bear to feel, and so has to be expelled. Also, this serves as a way in which the infant may feel unified with, or unseparated from caregivers. Because of the fantasy of non-separation, projective identification is a transitional form of relationship in which one feels alternately controlled by and in control of others. Naturally, these fantasies of non-separation and control continue through childhood and adolescence, into adult life and relationships.

Melanie Klein introduced projective identification in 1946 and discussed it in only one other paper, titled "On Identification" (1955/1984). But her protégé Wilfred Bion (1959) elaborated on the term and expanded its usage by demonstrating it to be an important interactive or communicative function between patient and therapist in individual therapy and the most powerful kind of unconscious communication in groups and couples. As Bion notably said: "The analyst feels that he is being manipulated so as to be playing a part, no matter how difficult to recognize, in somebody else's phantasy" (p. 149).

Bion described a certain kind of projective identification as a fantasy that expresses the desire to bring another person *under one's control* (cf., Gariepy-Boutin & Maas, 2017). This process typically goes back and forth between people, although it may also be one-sided. Bion also believed that projective identification is often accompanied by behavior designed to elicit in another *in reality* what the sender is, in fact, expelling or projecting through fantasy. For example, one person may project their experience of rage or rejection into another and then behave in such a way toward the other as to provoke such a state of rage or rejection in that other person. This is called *realistic projective identification*. Realistic projective identification plays an important role in what is known as "containment" in infancy when painful states of mind may be evoked in a parent by an agitated infant who will not be comforted. A good-enough parent will not retaliate in receiving a destructive or painful state of mind from the infant, but instead will "digest" the infant's experience and perhaps speak it back to them, as in: "You are really upset about that, aren't you?" Naturally, these early functions – projecting and identifying with another's state of mind – continue through all stages of development, into adult relationships.

Beyond Klein and Bion, other psychoanalysts who have used and developed projective identification as a clinical term and method of investigation include both Thomas Ogden and Donald Winnicott as well as Herbert Rosenfeld, Michael Balint, Harold Searles, Robert Caper, James Grotstein, and Polly Young-Eisendrath. These analysts have applied it variously to their clinical understanding of early development, psychotic process, unconscious communication, and couple or other close adult interpersonal relationships and intersubjective experiences.

Before Klein coined the term for preverbal communication between infant and mother, Carl Jung (1921/1971) came up with a similar idea in his book *Psychological Types*. Jung used the French term *participation mystique* (borrowed from the French ethnologist Lucien Levy-Bruhl) to denote a kind of collective psychological state or frame of mind in which the individual seems unable to keep the boundaries of individuality, but feels in partial identification with another or others. Jung used the term especially in regard to falling in love when one person feels convinced that they can experience exactly what the other is feeling and thinking – a conviction of a kind of emotional telepathy. Like Bion, Jung thought this kind of identification with another or others played a strong role in group psychology.

In the development and applications of the theory of projective identification, clinicians and theorists emphasize it as a link or channel between people that can produce or convey any or all of the following: direct communication "deeper" than words that involves our capacity to evoke emotional states and communicate our states of mind (Caper, 2000, 2020); the splitting of good/bad, life/death, internal/external, and ideal/devalued, which happens quickly and implicitly; the potential manipulation of another's psyche; fantasies of "clarity of insight" into another's "soul" that may or may not be reciprocated; and experiences of inexplicable danger, destruction, inflation, intoxication, or omnipotence. Truly, then, we can reference everything from falling in love to being terrified of a stranger, to being swept away with tears of gratitude with a spiritual teacher (even though you might not understand the words or language being spoken), to being taken in by the "charisma" of a despot. The clinical theory of projective identification maps a powerful communication that originates in our infancy. Ultimately, the theory tells us that projective identification cannot be rationalized or ignored in families, couples, and groups.

Projective identification in Dialogue Therapy

As we have said many times now, working through projective identification is the keystone of Dialogue Therapy, primarily through learning to use Real Dialogue as a skill, but also by partners gaining insight into one another's patterns and habits of projection and projective identification. Even during the couple's opening conversation for the Evaluation in the first meeting, Dialogue Therapists are looking to identify the particular patterns of projective identifications. The manner in which the dyad engages in the opening sequence of talking, and continues through the Evaluation, about why they have come and what they hope for, will begin to guide the therapists who are looking to make a map of the entangled dynamics of "doer and done-to" that are always presented by couples.

As mentioned earlier, we are always alert to the person who says: "Would you like to begin first?" That person *may* be directing the other in a way that is pressured and confusing. The ways in which the second person responds (whether automatically carrying out the "command" to begin, raising a question, hesitating, or turning the tables) will say something about the push–pull of projective identification in this particular pair. Answering the Six Questions (see Chapter 6), talking about the ways in which each partner perceives "the problems in the relationship," and then completing the Relational History, will open up the entire psychological theater of what the partners are unconsciously playing out.

The drama of projective identification

Take, for example, Bill and Kathy[1] – a couple we will be describing throughout this book. It was clear from the beginning that Kathy was the partner to "be believed" in their relationship. Kathy's concerns, presented from the start, were about "how to make our relationship more delightful, but," she said, she sometimes felt "it lacked oomph." When Bill began to speak, it was clear that *he lacked* oomph, which was partly due to his 40-hours-per-week delivery job, followed every day by making dinner for him and Kathy. Kathy, on the other hand, did not have a job (although she sometimes taught a class), and she implied and conveyed explicitly that she was "aligned with the Universe" so that she could "decide according to my wishes and freedom" what "I will and will not do." Unmentioned by either of them, but discovered in her Relational History, Kathy continued to be partly financially supported by her parents in her adult life, given what she needed when she asked, especially by her father. Thus, Kathy did not have to work in order to earn a living to support herself, and could be "free" of such daily obligations as Bill had.

So, the projective identification looked like this: Bill idealized Kathy and her freedom while diminishing himself for not being able to "align with the Universe" and working a job he didn't like. Kathy also implied that Bill "just didn't get how to do the metaphysics of universal alignment." Additionally, Kathy's father, who is a doctor, was "angry all the time about his work," and Kathy just didn't see the point of all that work. Bill, on the other hand, was very tired, self-defeating, and yes, angry (in a passive aggressive way) that he couldn't bring about what Kathy wanted. When Bill asked Kathy to help with the dishes after he cooked, she said she would "do that only when it fits my schedule and desires, because my freedom is more important to me than anything else." Kathy unconsciously diminished and dismissed Bill, and he unconsciously identified with that. And they both idealized Kathy. In the unconscious split, Kathy was supposed to bring "all things" to the couple and allow Bill to pursue his art (they are also both artists) while "showing" him how to do "the right metaphysics." Within the projective identification: Kathy is a goddess and Bill is a lump. Bill's lumpiness irritated Kathy because she felt that he often didn't express himself or show his own initiative. Bill couldn't "understand" why he was stuck in his lump, so to speak. There is more to their story, but this projective identification created the unconscious barrier to them making a serious decision: whether to adopt a child or to use infertility services; for while they were trying to get Kathy pregnant, it was discovered through medical evaluation that Bill is infertile. They found they would simply get "bogged down" in conversations about "freedom" when they faced their decision-making, although both said they wanted to be parents.

Dialogue Therapists get used to picking up on the unconscious themes of projective identification. One such theme is the *zero-sum game*: in the couple it seems only one person can either thrive or win or succeed. Or, each person feels that "the other one" has more options and more possibilities. Within the zero-sum mentality of projective identification is often a "life-death" theme. Here is a clear example: Andrea grew up in a Jewish family in which her parents were survivors of the Holocaust, and she felt that she "was never allowed to suffer or have serious problems" because "my life was supposed to be *wonderful!*" And now she is married to Kim[2] who found out only a few years ago that she

(Kim) has a chronic immune system disorder that requires elaborate planning and preparations regarding food, cleanliness, and health concerns. They also have a son, Alex, who is ten years old and attends a private school more than five miles from where they live. The presenting issues had to do with the fact that Kim felt that Andrea was not doing her part in helping with the responsibilities of getting Alex ready and to school in the mornings. Kim felt that this was threatening her health. Andrea is the greater breadwinner, and she needs to get up early for her work and get to her computer, even before Alex leaves the house. Kim has a part-time job, but she also works hard on composing music and is somewhat successful as a musician and singer.

Within the projective identification, Andrea feels "completely trapped in Kim's illness" as though "I don't have a right to have my own suffering or misery because only *hers* counts." And Kim says, "I *always* had to give up my own needs in my family of origin where I was the youngest sister of three; *the others* got their needs met while my parents were young and successful. My parents divorced when I was in middle school and I always felt that only the 'successful' ones counted – my older sisters. Now, it's the same with Andrea because *she* makes more money." For Andrea, it seemed that she was caught in the "life-death threat" of Kim's illness where she, Andrea, "couldn't hold a candle to that threat." (It was like having parents who suffered through the Holocaust compared to her "regular" suffering in childhood, Andrea reflected.) And Kim agreed that her illness was a life-death drama: "I actually *know* that I won't live a full lifetime unless I take care of myself *now*." It seemed as though there was no space for either partner: Andrea, because she felt she couldn't deny Kim the support she needed; and Kim, because she felt she couldn't live in the current conditions. Finally, Andrea said: "Why should I even try to talk to her about the mornings? I don't have a card to play in the game; she always wins." Neither one felt they had "room to breathe"; Andrea felt she could not allow herself to have legitimate needs, and Kim felt she couldn't breathe if she didn't get support with Alex, their son.

Another theme of zero-sum is often about who is more desirable, attractive, interesting, or compelling of the partners. Again, there is a sense that there can be only one such person in the couple and the other one *has* to be "just not as compelling." So let's think about Bella and Jack who came to Dialogue Therapy because they "no longer have a sex life." They had "already tried polyamory; but it just made everything more complicated." Now in their early forties, they had met in the mountains of Chile when they were in their late twenties, both of them trekking around, having an "amazing and wonderful life" and feeling like – "boom, I just met my soul mate!" According to Bella, Jack "was hot and lots of women and men wanted to sleep with him." She was proud that she "landed him" and felt that having done so "proved something about her own sexiness." Bella has always seen herself as "too big" in both her physical and her psychological attributes. She thought she was "big-boned" and "more handsome than beautiful" and had "too much of a mouth along with too much of a brain." Bella had graduated with degrees in Physics and Philosophy from an elite college, but then "couldn't find her dream" afterward. So she went trekking. Jack made her "feel like a woman, more feminine," and he "seemed excited about my mind." When Jack and Bella were first together they were the envy of everyone. Each thought the other was the most attractive creature who ever lived. They were each other's "trophy partner."

Once they married, though, Bella wanted to go to graduate school and pursue a career in science. They also decided "late" to have Lily, who was now just two years old. And Bella now felt like her appearance had become "shabby compared to my twenties," and that Jack "still has all of his charms and looks." Bella was in graduate school, working hard to finish projects while Jack was working a full-time tech job at home. Jack was the "nanny" for Lily, and Bella complained that "Lily just *loves him more*, and he gets all of the really sweet awake hours with her." Bella believed that the changes in her appearance due to aging and childbirth were the reasons that Jack "was pulling away sexually."

Jack said he was "just tired all of the time," and that he felt "undervalued" by Bella; she didn't seem grateful that he was taking care of Lily so that she, Bella, could go to grad school. In fact, Jack rarely approached her for intimacy. Because their athleticism and good looks had been so important to both of them in their courtship and early marriage, it now seemed that their lack of intimacy and feelings of alienation must be related to their appearances.

Bella thought she'd just lost her appeal, while Jack thought that she "wasn't attracted to *him* anymore" because she never expressed gratitude or concern for his feelings, even though she would try to have sex with him. Jack felt that he was "just too tired" to have sex, and thought that, because he "rarely got a chance to go out for a run," he lacked libido. Neither of them felt their partner was attracted and both felt deeply rejected. The initial idealization of the partner had now turned to envy of the other's "special circumstances" and the belief that they were "stuck with someone" who would never love them.

Projective identification can also take the form of a *hall of mirrors* such as the following case in which each partner felt invalidated and alienated from the other's friends and colleagues. Devan came to the first session of Dialogue Therapy with a tearful complaint that her husband Kendal "never seems interested in my faith or what I want to share from my many deepest spiritual experiences."

Devan is a Jehovah's Witness who takes her religion to heart. She is active in the church community and believes that everything good within her has been strengthened by having become a Witness, just five years before. She is thirty-five years old and has one child with Kendal. Kendal, thirty-six, is Rastafarian, although he doesn't feel it's exactly his religion, more his "lifestyle."

Devan and Kendal, in the opening conversation, both mentioned how happy they are to be together and how much their relationship means to them. But Devan admitted that she feels as though "Kendal devalues me, and puts me down, because I am a Jehovah's Witness." She said she often feels that he is making fun of her beliefs or just not interested, and she worries that he "doesn't have a *true spiritual path*." Kendal said that he is "fine" with her religion, but doesn't want her "trying to download it into me," and that he is sometimes worried "my wife is in a cult."

Both people feel diminished for their beliefs by the other (and a little embarrassed by the other's beliefs), and it seems that they cannot stop talking about these "spiritual" issues that undermine their sense of friendship and pride in being good parents. Devan also reacts to Kendal's criticism that her religion is a "cult." Many of her friends are Jehovah's Witnesses, and she feels uncomfortable bringing them to her home because of her husband's reactions. Similarly, Kendal doesn't like hanging out with his Rasta friends around Devan because "she always seems to feel like her ways of doing things are *just better* than mine." When Devan and Kendal talk about their feelings of humiliation and hurt, and about their spiritual beliefs, it seems they are in a crazy hall of mirrors in which each one says almost exactly the same things the other one says. It seems impossible to know who is doing what to whom. This is typical of some forms of projective identification.

Untangling projective identifications in Dialogue Therapy

There are steps in the process of Dialogue Therapy for untangling, naming, and describing the projective identifications of each individual. In later chapters, we will give details of how this process works. But here, we outline the steps with some examples and illustrations from the couple, Bill and Kathy. (See Appendix A for the Evaluation and Relational History templates.)

First, in completing the Six Questions as part of the Evaluation, Bill and Kathy present a kind of hall-of-mirrors theme in which each of them is anxious about their individual freedom: Kathy believes that Bill doesn't really know how to work with their shared *metaphysical* approach to "get his needs met," and consequently, Bill "does a job that he doesn't *want* to do" (Bill agrees with this). Meanwhile, Kathy feels very strongly that she "needs to make her own decisions about freedom," and together they agree that questions about how they divide up chores and care for themselves (their freedom) are troubling both of them. They also know that becoming parents "limits freedom." They both agree that Bill is a "lump" and Kathy is a "goddess." And they agree that you have to align "with the universe" in order to get your needs met. But they can't make important decisions together.

Second, in talking together about their answers to the Six Questions (described in Chapter 6), Bill and Kathy talk about their problems around decision-making and protecting their free time. Therapists are listening for the tangles of "the doer/done-to" mentality in terms of zero-sum or hall-of-mirrors themes or something else about "who is doing what to whom."

And finally, in the Relational History part of the Evaluation, therapists are listening for repeated phrases, images, and feelings during each partner's falling in love and later disillusionment in this and their earlier committed relationships. The Dialogue Therapist is listening for those same phrases, images, and feelings in regard to one or both parents and/or siblings. Typically, these themes and phrases will be identical or clear. For Kathy, the repeated themes involved her father and Bill doing "work they dislike" and how Kathy feels close to her father "when he gives me what I want" (and how, in her view, Bill has not been able to do that). Kathy also idealizes her suburban childhood and her mother's freedom to "do what she wanted to do with her life." Bill, on the other hand, idealizes his parents' commitment to the principles and values related to living in an intentional community where they spent their adult lives. Bill also seemed to have unquestioned faith in "Kathy's wisdom" just as he also had faith in his parents' wisdom and authority.

By the conclusion of the Evaluation, Dialogue Therapists will have formulated some kind of map or framework for how each partner is stepping into a projective identification that repeats aspects of early development and how that process is defensive and/or re-traumatizing.

This formulation is typically presented to the partners in the Wrap-Up at the end of the Evaluation (see Chapter 9 for examples of Wrap-Up). It goes something like this: "Bill, you have had a tendency to idealize Kathy in just the ways you idealized your parents, whereby you see her as providing the 'wisdom' for the two of you. You also then feel afraid to tell her directly your needs, desires, and complaints; you seem afraid to have conflicts with her. Consequently, you don't stand up for yourself and speak to Kathy like an adult. This is very frustrating for her, and obstructs her view of you as a man, a mature adult who is fully responsible for his life, and is capable of sharing *his* wisdom with others (e.g., a child). Your idealization of Kathy keeps you from telling her directly, for example, that you want to become a father." And then: "Kathy, you receive Bill's idealization with a self-affirmation of your 'greater wisdom,' even though you would like him to 'man-up.' You don't like to see him disappear into the background, but you also don't seem to acknowledge how much he adds to your life through his work and other contributions. You tend to idealize your father for giving you what you want, and to assume that Bill can't do that – because he does not have personal wealth, nor aspire to it. You also idealize the state of 'being free' as though you fear that carrying responsibilities in your everyday life automatically erases all your freedom."

The map of projective identifications is used by the therapist within the sessions of Dialogue Therapy, both in terms of outlining the emotional habits, triggers, and obstacles, and, in terms of reflecting on situations that require Unblocking (see Chapter 8 for details on Unblocking). Unblocking is a mini "individual therapy session" with one partner (with the other partner observing) that takes place when the Dialogue Therapist switches chairs with one person and works on a particular obstacle that is blocking the process of using Real Dialogue or interfering with the therapist's ability to Facilitate, Coach, or act as an Alter-Ego.

Throughout the course of Dialogue Therapy, the therapist refers to the map of projective identifications for each partner when Real Dialogue breaks down. By the end of a successful DT treatment, each partner will have a fairly clear sense of the dynamics and motivations of their own projective identifications and will know how to step back from them. Also, each partner will recognize their own vulnerabilities, as well as those of the other, expressed in the emotional patterns and limitations that have carried over from childhood dynamics. Projective identification thus plays a central role at all levels of Dialogue Therapy. As we move through the chapters on set-up, techniques and methods of Dialogue Therapy and Real Dialogue, the uses of projective identification will be further illuminated. We will see how Dialogue Therapists help partners to create a mindful gap between them so that they can become differentiated individuals who can then maintain an emotional space in which to be curious and intimate as partners.

Notes

1 We have permission to use any and all of the recorded materials of Dialogue Therapy with this couple (Bill and Kathy) for educational purposes.

2 All references to partners and couples other than Bill and Kathy have been disguised and are collages of couples in Dialogue Therapy.

Bibliography

Bion, W. (1959). *Experiences in Groups*. New York: Basic Books.

Caper, R. (2000). *Immaterial Facts: Freud's Discovery of Psychic Reality and Klein's Development of His Work*. London: Routledge.

Gariepy-Boutin, C. & Maas, K. (2017). "Emprise et satisfaction: the theory of Paul Denis." *Presentation at Vermont Association for Psychoanalytic Studies Annual Meeting*, Burlington, VT.

Jung, C. (1921/1971). *Psychological Types: Collected Works, Volume 6*. Princeton, NJ: Princeton University Press.

Klein, M. (1984). *Envy and Gratitude and Other Works: 1946–1963*. London: Hogarth Press.

Ogden, T. (1991). *Projective Identification and Psychotherapeutic Technique*. Northvale, NJ: Jason Aronson.

Winnicott, D. (1956). "Primary maternal preoccupation." *Collected Papers: Through Paediatrics to Psychoanalysis* (pp. 300–305). London: Tavistock Publications.

4 The "be-attitudes" for therapists and couples in Dialogue Therapy

Given that projective identification creates an emotionally charged interpersonal environment, effective couple therapy warrants a highly structured contained engagement with clients. In this chapter, we set the stage for the emotional tone and attitudes that Dialogue Therapists will assume within themselves and with their clients, as they enter into a process of Evaluation, inquiry, reflecting, Coaching, Facilitating, Alter-Ego/Doubling, and Unblocking. These are the suggested "ways to be," or what we call the "be-attitudes," when doing Dialogue Therapy. They require both a kind of equanimity (matter-of-fact, evenly distributed attention) and a knowledge of DT methods and theory.

Young-Eisendrath (1984) espouses two important attitudes for Dialogue Therapists: *informed discovery* and *objective empathy*. Informed discovery is an attitude of openness whereby the therapists bring conscious plans, ideas, and knowledge into the therapeutic relationship, but hold them tentatively, in the spirit of discovery. Informed discovery is "an attitude of mind that permits one to see through confusion to understanding, to see through the facts to the truth" (p. 107). This attitude depends on being comfortable enough with one's training and clinical orientation to hold them lightly, with humor and humility, permitting the advantage of what Symington (1993) calls *creative action* in the clinical moment, or again, Winnicott's (1957/1992) *potential space* or *play space*.

Once clinicians have completed their DT training and have had some experience through which they increase their ease with the method, the structured nature of Dialogue Therapy often allows them to hold more lightly their clinical tasks. After practicing the entire sequence of sessions with ten to fifteen couples, accompanied by conversations with experienced Dialogue Therapists, as well as with a clinical consultation group, the Dialogue Therapist feels confident and at ease in many sessions. When that level of expertise has been achieved, the be-attitudes are more easily applied.

Objective empathy, the second be-attitude in the therapist, is a natural outgrowth of insight and equanimity born of the study of the self, as well as other kinds of personal development, including the therapist's personal psychotherapy (strongly recommended for Dialogue Therapists), formal education, and living a full life. This kind of empathy requires allowing a tension within oneself (therapist) between "feeling intuitively into" an individual or a couple, and

DOI: 10.4324/9781003200840-4

making clinical assessments, while holding one's own *subjectivity* as a studied awareness. Slochower (1996) refers to this type of holding as "bracketing" – that is, acknowledging one's own personality, with its limitations and complexes, without indulging those complexes or emotional reactions. As a term, objective empathy points to our ability to inquire between self and other long enough to grasp the other's pain and emotional meaning, and even "feel into" them, while also being able to return to one's own mind and a fluid thinking process. Therapists and counselors may sometimes be swept up into a flood of feeling or a narrative that leads to *identifying with* one of the partners or even with both, and then believing the stories about who "did what to whom."

Couples coming into therapy always have stories of shame and blame. In Dialogue Therapy, it is especially important to take a step back from partners' narratives and really know the distinction between empathy and identification. Whereas empathy allows us to "step into" another's experience or another's world while holding onto our own, identification leaves us feeling as though we directly *know* another's experience and find ourselves acting on this assumption. In Dialogue Therapy, we are expected to have an "objective" attitude (i.e., to be able to stand back and study our experiences and our thoughts) alongside our concern and caring, and to use our empathy in a more clinical manner than in some other kinds of couple therapy. For example, Emotion-Focused Therapy (EFT) reportedly depends on a warmly engaged therapist with whom partners are meant to have a "positive transference." In DT, partners are meant to feel like they are with "an expert whom they can trust," even in the midst of their worst and most dangerous aggressive or destructive feelings. Other therapeutic terms for objective empathy might be "mentalization" (Fonagy, Gyorgy, Jurist, & Target, 2004) or "social metacognition" (Flavell, 1979; Briñol & DeMaree, 2012).

Dialogue Therapists cultivate objective empathy especially when they engage as Alter-Egos with one of the partners. At such times, Dialogue Therapists temporarily "step into" the subjective experience of one of the partners and try putting into words what is intuitively sensed by combining observation and the therapist's "feeling into" moods, impressions, and implications. This process overlaps with the practice of "using one's countertransference experiences," as it's called in psychoanalytic therapy, to create and try out a language that clients might use to understand their emotional lives and experiences. In a certain way, Alter-Ego work is like "method acting": one steps into the character of the partner through both observations and intuitions, and makes a guess about how to express *what is not being expressed* or is being implied or used in an attack on the partner.[1]

Over the course of Dialogue Therapy, partners will also be encouraged to develop their own objective empathy with each other, especially in times of conflict, through their attempts to understand the partner's implied and unspoken experiences. The session called Role Reversal is designed to assess what partners have intuited empathically about each other through the DT process.

Pressures of projective identification on the Dialogue Therapist

As we described in Chapter 3, a major impact of projective identification is feeling kidnapped into another's emotional experiences. Instead of empathy, this invites the desire to identify with the other's experiences, manage the other person emotionally, or even control the other's behaviors. When projective identification is *idealizing*, as in falling in love, emotional kidnapping can be intoxicating, as partners "fall into" each other's desires. Typically, falling in love is embraced as wholly positive at the beginning of a romantic relationship. But when idealizations invert – as they must – this inversion is often characterized by *negativity* or *hostility* that lead to the *disillusionment* phase of the romance. Then, chronic hostile and destructive projective identifications (as in the zero-sum game) deaden the couple's vitality. Conflicts become repetitive and emotionally threatening and trust is gradually eroded. In this kind of unconscious communication, partners feel compelled to see, hear, and feel things in a particular way, as though there were no freedom of choice. The belief, then, is that "*the other person is making me 'be' or 'feel' this way.*" When partners' communications are consumed by chronic projective identification, emotional threat levels can remain acute and crippling to both people, and alternatives seem to be unknown.

Given this situation, Dialogue Therapists approach their work with an awareness of the pressures on them to trigger their own projective identifications vis-à-vis either of the partners or the couple as a whole. Recognizing and accurately mapping the couple's projective identifications require informed discovery and objective empathy – and therefore stepping back from entering into a projective identification with either partner. And so, interpretations are addressed mostly to what partners are doing *with each other*, not what either partner is doing with the therapist.

The focus on individuals: no secrets, no blame

While we understand and subscribe to the notion that *the couple* is our "client," and that the relationship itself is a type of "third element" that is more than the sum of its parts, we also strongly underscore the fact that the *two individuals* in the couple have their own particular cultural backgrounds, emotional histories, life experiences, dreams, fantasies, values, aesthetics, bodies, and ideal selves. Being a couple can never accommodate all these differences, nor does anyone come to the relationship with all the skills needed to cope with unconscious dynamics. The emotional meanings of one partner's language may not have any inherent resonance for the other partner, but the interpersonal field nonetheless organizes itself around the assumptions and meanings each partner *creates* about the other. These creations become reified in such a way that certain aspects of the individuals are *provoked, evoked,* and *invoked* in repetitive and rigid ways.

When couples are trapped in chronic negative projective identifications, we often hear them say things like, "That's just the way you are, and you're never going to change" or "You *always* do it that way." It is as though a temporary state has hardened into a permanent trait – except, they may notice that that "trait" doesn't seem to be present when their partner is with someone else – say, a friend or another relative. When the two separate individual subjectivities, with their own psychological and emotional meanings, are not addressed in couple therapy, the emotional pressures and desires driving partners cannot be tracked and hence the problematic unconscious patterns continue even after couple therapy seems to have been "helpful." In Dialogue Therapy, we regard the "self" as an *interactive process* (comprising internal fantasies and external expressions) and encourage curiosity in ourselves and in the couple about each individual's meaning-making or interpretive approaches.

Within the guidelines of objective empathy, the Dialogue Therapist fosters a "no-fault" atmosphere for and about the couple. When partners trust that no one will be blamed, the likelihood of honest self-disclosure increases and some of the typical obstructions to engaging in therapy dissolve. One frequent example, writes Young-Eisendrath (1984), rife with potential for negative expectations and judgments is "the speaking of secrets":

> Once we have intuited or otherwise discovered a secret is being kept from one partner (usually involving a sexual or financial betrayal), we do everything we can to encourage the secret to come forth . . . [We talk] about the 'magic binding' power of secrets to isolate the partners from each other . . . basic trust [is] a flame which can die out if it does not have proper tending and adequate fuel and air. Secrets tend to stifle the flame.
>
> (p. 121)

Naturally, Dialogue Therapists understand that privacy and secrecy are different in important ways, and that each partner needs a private life of the mind while still being a part of a couple. It is only when a secret eclipses an intimate connection to one's partner, and poses a threat to relationship commitment, that we treat it as problematic and as a matter for Real Dialogue.

Given that we proceed with a no-blame policy, Dialogue Therapists handle *all interviews* with both partners present together in the room. When one partner is interviewed, the other sits behind, out of the field of vision of the interviewee. In this way, there is no secret-keeping about the other partner in a separate interview. Dialogue Therapists approach this work with other crucial attitudes that are meant to telegraph and enhance the sense of safety, hope, and engagement in dialogue for the couple. These attitudes include mindfulness, Witnessing, and what Young-Eisendrath (2019) calls the "Three Cs": commitment, constraint, and containment. While the "Three Cs" are capacities that the therapists hope to strengthen in the partners, the C's are also important for the therapists to model.

Commitment

Commitment to each other, including the therapists to the couple, is the first pillar of a secure therapy process in Dialogue Therapy. The therapist, having taken on the couple, is committed to the DT method in its structure and aims, and demonstrates this commitment by adhering to the method and themes of the DT sessions – within reasonable limits. Dialogue Therapy sessions are described to the couple in written form (either hard copy or digital) or over the telephone before the couple enters the first meeting. Having understood the general parameters of DT, the couple gives informed consent to go through the process.

Because the Evaluation *precedes* the actual DT sessions, and yet is *part of* the process, the couple needs to see and comprehend the overview of the entire process *before* entering into the first meeting. And so, couples should be informed that the Evaluation is the first step in the therapy, but an important decision is made at its Wrap-Up: whether continuing the DT process to its conclusion would be therapeutic or helpful for that particular couple. (More information on the Evaluation is presented in Chapter 6.)

And finally, in the most promising cases, partners are able to say at the outset of the therapy that they are committed to each other and their relationship. In other words, DT is about *improving* committed relationships. Of course, DT deals with partners who have lost their faith and trust in their relationship, or who are new at their relationship and are concerned to do their best with it. And yet the Dialogue Therapist lets partners know, even from the first meeting, that the therapy is most effective for partners who are committed to each other. Typically, partners are also expected to have made a "home" for their relationship – either living together or living in some arrangement that supports it – at least by the conclusion of the DT process.

Constraint

Heidegger (1962) wrote of the "thrown-ness" or "thrown-in-ness" (*Geworfen*) of our lives, of our bodies, and geography, and of our family circumstances and historical cohort. We don't control or choose most of our circumstances in life. Rather, we are thrown into them and must "show up," even though we have not chosen them. These constraints confront us with the issues of acceptance and of embracing the limitations of our humanity, the environment, and ourselves (Inwood, 1999). As we work on ourselves to retain a sense of gentle matter-of-factness before we decide how we want to communicate or act, we have greater freedom to do what seems to be constructive and creative. We don't like the limitations (e.g., that we die) and constraints (e.g., that we age) of our lives, but we must work with them, all the same. We are always and in everything constrained.

There are constraints that come from without and those that come from within. Within ourselves we have a degree of freedom if we can restrain our emotional reactivity so that we may change our attitude, our perspective, or our point of view on the realities we face. Young-Eisendrath (2019) views the struggle with constraint as a spiritual and existential task – a type of work that asks us to find meaning in our limitations. Given DT's constraints and structure, we ask therapists and the couple to use a form of restraint, a thoughtful inhibition of their most impulsive, hurtful, raw, or brute reactions, at least while in the consulting room.

Embracing a path of constraint or restraint goes against many contemporary movements or ideals (like the value of expressing one's rage) that seem not to understand the importance of constraint. In many North American societies right now, our opinions, criticisms, judgments, or contempt, in their raw forms, drop out of our mouths like so much candy from a gum ball machine. This type of impulsive speech and action tends to create a repetitive interaction or cycle of attack and defense (humiliation-rage) that can seem unstoppable once it gets underway. Dialogue Therapy requires that all parties in the consulting room lower the level of emotional threat.

Dialogue Therapists are trained to coach the partners away from raw attacks on each other and destructive acting out (for example, jumping up and running out of the consulting room). The therapists are also trained to stop aggressive attacks from one partner on the other or on the therapist, even in the opening conversation, if they appear to be humiliating or enraging.

In these kinds of enactments, we all "lose our minds" when the mindful gap is obliterated. Therapists and partners are encouraged not to lose their minds in the consulting room, but instead to use the skills of Real Dialogue. Therapists model these skills even before the partners learn them. Therapists also show the partners that they can pause or wait in order to speak. One of the most helpful utterances people can offer may be something like, "I'd like to think about that for a minute before I say more" or "Help me understand what you mean when you say that." In fact, Pieniadz often quips that partners should carry around a laminated card (like those used in some cognitive-behavioral programs) which they can consult at tense moments, that has stock phrases that help create a mindful gap to constrain their impulses to attack and defend. From the first moment they communicate with clients, Dialogue Therapists are expected to use RD skills every step of the way. Constraint and restraint remind us to accept our situation in order to understand it and decide *how we want to respond*, instead of pushing and pulling on ourselves or others in ways that are destructive.

Containment

Containment is an ability to keep hostile or harmful impulses under control. Containment develops from accepting the reality of the necessary constraints in our lives. Emotional containment includes our ability to reflect on the possible consequences of our actions *before* those actions are taken, so as to evaluate them and apply boundaries around them, or to transform them into respectful and lov-ing ways of relating (Young-Eisendrath, 2019). To paraphrase Freud, we are able to send our thoughts and imagination out ahead of us, almost as a reconnaissance party or as what he called "experimental action," before we actually say or do something that may cause damage by not being able to be retracted. Containment is a type of "holding" or "bracketing" of our first impulse in order to find a mindful space from which to respond (Slochower, 1996).

Dialogue Therapists model this behavior by not reacting too dramatically or sentimentally to the reports that partners bring to the therapeutic table. Dialogue Therapists calmly repeat, query, interpret, or instruct – as when they are adjusting the couple's language when acting as Alter-Egos while encouraging partners to approach the dialogue similarly. Young-Eisendrath (2019) states:

> If you can recognize your own feelings and not take them to be the final word on reality, then you can step back in times of agitation and reflect on what you want to do or say . . . [T]here is a secret weapon in this process, one that we all have a hard time embracing: *Don't take things too personally* . . . [Y]ou have to expand your capacity to not take on what is not yours and to distinguish between what you are responsible for and what simply happens.
>
> (p. 78)

Incidentally, and paradoxically, not taking things personally is one of the most "efficient" routes to actually *experiencing* what is one's own personal psychology and what isn't. Containment buys enough space and time to allow a genuine thinking process to occur and meaningful psychic connections to be made (Bion, 1959). Such connections, in their turn, create more breathing room, more freedom for individuals to be themselves and appreciate their partners' unique selves.

We also know it is merely aspirational, and not always possible (especially early in the DT process, but also a lifelong challenge) to hesitate and bracket one's raw reactions or contain oneself. Nevertheless, containment is a practice in which we attempt to hold our experiences in mind long enough to reflect on them – even if something hurtful *has already* been said. If there has been a painful exchange, then we can revisit it in dialogue. This reflection and revisiting ("You know, I've been thinking about something you said, and I would like to talk more about it") demonstrate that the importance of the partner and the relationship has been held in mind even through the painful events.

The be-attitudes of informed discovery and objective empathy are cultivated by Dialogue Therapists and in the practice of Real Dialogue through a contained emotional response to what partners present. These attitudes mean that it will be the conscious intention of Dialogue Therapists not to align emotionally with either partner.

A be-attitude about the uses of transference/countertransference in Dialogue Therapy

As Dialogue Therapists help partners understand the historical dynamics, trauma, wounding, and emotional repetitions enacted with the other partner, they interpret and point out the "re-transcription" of earlier emotional relating onto the current interchange. In this way, working through the dynamics of projective identification is similar to working through these dynamics in all forms of analytic therapy in which the therapist and patient constitute a shared field of unconscious communication. In DT, partners have to do the work of grieving, i.e., recognizing what has been lost as a result of their projective identifications, and how self and partner could not and cannot be otherwise. The grief work in DT is aimed at realizing that neither self nor partner can be the fantasy or the idealized figure that one longs for, and that important opportunities may have already been lost as a result of destructive relational patterns (Stern, 1997). The focus of understanding and grieving lost opportunities is always a part of couple relationship. Interventions that help the partners in DT are discovered and processed within this interactive field; as partners learn to truly dialogue with each other, their transferences *to each other* are altered.

Different from many other couple therapies, Dialogue Therapy conveys a sense of order and structure and containment from the start. Chaotic and disruptive attacks from either partner to the other, or onto the therapist, are interrupted even early in the process (and at any time thereafter) and redirected. As much as possible, hostile enactments are prevented from taking place in the consulting room. There is also no first session in which the therapist seems to be groping around to understand the problems or manage the couple's enactments. Instead, the first session is a series of tasks that immediately reveal a variety of emotional patterns and issues between partners.

Because of the structure and efficiency of the set-up, there can be an immediate idealizing transference directed at the therapist. Or, potentially, there can be a negative transference because a Dialogue Therapist will repeatedly direct partners back to the tasks at hand. No matter which way the transference may go, the Dialogue Therapist responds as much as possible with a neutral, businesslike attitude. Only on rare occasions does a Dialogue Therapist interpret transference to the therapeutic relationship or to the set-up in order to restore the DT process.

We do not generally view partners or their relationship as "broken" or "pathological," as much as needing understanding and acceptance of various de-idealizations, in order to make room for their real, imperfect, and potentially surprising life together. In this way, Dialogue Therapy resembles most other forms of therapy and analysis: it aims to help clients confront reality and turn away from idealizations that are costly to their sense of trust in each other and their fully-lived lives. The DT process involves the therapist(s) being able to "court surprise," as Stern (1997) says, thereby encouraging the partners to do the same for each other. As Perel (2006) has noted, the possibility that there are still many things to know, i.e., to *not assume*, about one's partner makes for excitement and desire in the relationship.

The balance and movement between knowing and not knowing, for a Dialogue Therapist, is a little bit tightrope and a little bit trapeze, and not really as dangerous as either of these. Dialogue Therapists bring the safety nets of open-heartedness, humor, creativity, and equanimity to each session and express these attributes especially during the Wrap-Up at the end. In the co-therapy model, co-therapists express this kind of open inquiry with each other in their interchanges about what they witness in the couple when speaking as a Reflecting Team. In the solo model, the individual Dialogue Therapist conveys the be-attitudes of informed discovery and objective empathy, especially at the end of each session in reporting to the couple about what the therapist has been thinking, seeing, and hearing during the session.

When the Dialogue Therapist reacts with equanimity and objective empathy to a couple's thinly veiled panic at various stages, especially at the beginning (which is quite common and understandable), partners immediately tend to relax. And then, when the couple sees the structure and process of the Evaluation and the Real Dialogue sessions – as well as the ordinariness in therapists' responses to the stresses and crises reported by partners – a greater ease develops between even the most distressed or hostile partners.

It is hard to overstate the relief that many partners feel when their worst and most negative enactments can be understood and digested rather quickly and expertly. Many Dialogue Therapy sessions include dialogue about what may have seemed to be unspeakable betrayals, threats, and losses. These aspects of the couple's history often come forward quickly during the Evaluation. The be-attitudes give partners hope and relief, and allow the Dialogue Therapists to gain confidence rather quickly in working with even the most difficult couples.

Mindfulness and the be-attitudes in Dialogue Therapy practice and training

Mindfulness is a conscious attempt to cultivate a kind of awareness that is both alert and concentrated, as well as relaxed and gentle or matter-of-fact. Mindfulness practices range from meditation to other practices (like Real Dialogue) that ask us to constrain our impulses and focus instead on our state of mind. When we are responding mindfully to any experience, we combine concentration and equanimity. This means we can pay close attention (through senses) and tolerate or remain open to our experiences, even when they are jarring or painful. Mindfulness practices cultivate our ability to accept constraints, not to push and pull on our experiences while they are happening, and to contain our impulses through various kinds of techniques, including focusing on an object of concentration, such as the breath or the words and meaning of one's partner. This kind of attitude is exactly what Freud (1955) called "evenly hovering attention," or the kind of attention that does not sharply veer toward or away from experiences, but allows experiences to unfold.

In training to become a Dialogue Therapist, all trainees learn how to do a simple mindfulness meditation called *Seeing Out and Seeing In*, *Hearing Out and Hearing In*, and *Feeling Out and Feeling In*. This practice focuses on our ordinary subjective experience of seeing "the world out there" and "images in the mind's eye"; hearing the sounds and words that are "coming from others," and hearing "the talking in one's own head"; and feeling the sensations of the body that form a "boundary between self and world," as well as the emotions "inside the body."[2]

During and after the training, Dialogue Therapists are encouraged to practice this meditation until they have developed some facility in tracking their own subjective experiences *in vivo* – something called *knowing your own snow globe*. In the language of DT, our subjective world is labeled a *snow globe*, enclosed within itself and readily shaken up. Each snow globe is a distinct world, different from others. The radical subjectivity of individual human perception and cognition is well established through research in cognitive science (see, e.g., Hoffman, 2019). Similarly, studies of eye witnesses (e.g., Loftus, 1979) and of prejudice and bias (e.g., Banaji & Greenwald, 2016) also demonstrate the gaps between what we believe we perceive and what we actually perceive. Our human condition of radical subjectivity means that there is very little possible consensus between adults about what they see, hear, and feel. Naturally, we have feelings of isolation and want to be witnessed! Otherwise, we may feel alienated and alone, anathema for the social beings we are. As we sharpen our abilities to perceive our own experiences distinctly, we can speak more precisely about them, and hence share them without arguing with others.

In general, mindfulness as a meditation or communication practice increases our concentration and equanimity, leading to greater clarity of perception. Developing the skills of Real Dialogue is a mindfulness practice. Speaking for Yourself, for example, requires being engaged with the specificity of one's own subjectivity. We each have our own memories, desires, feelings, opinions, aches, and pains, and other people do not have access to accurate perceptions of them without our words. Many triggers for negative projections and projective identifications come from this universal condition of our individual subjectivity. From the time of early childhood, we are encouraged to "use your words, not your actions" to communicate with others (e.g., "Don't hit your brother – tell him you are angry!"). But we also notice how our words repeatedly fail to get across our emotional states, desires, hurts, etc. to others. When it comes to an intimate partner, we feel that that person, above all, "should just know" what we are trying to convey in our words and gestures. Inevitably, that person fails and we feel humiliated, rejected, spurned, or enraged.

During the actual Dialogue Therapy sessions, mindfulness is cultivated through learning and practicing the skills called *Real Dialogue*. These three skills are described next. The three booklets offered to clients and therapists-in-training that illustrate the meaning and philosophy of these skills of Real Dialogue are presented in full in Appendix B. The two additional capacities then described – *Responding* and *Witnessing* – fill out the picture of what is cultivated through the interpersonal mindfulness of RD. First, the skills of RD:

1   *Speaking for Yourself* encourages us to wake up to a personal responsibility to speak in a subjective manner in order to lower the emotional threat level when we are involved in respectful and skillful conflict. Of course,

it asks us to use only "I-statements" and no "We" or "You" statements. But that is just the beginning. This skill requires us to experience and take responsibility for the fact that the other person cannot know (i.e., cannot read minds) or even precisely feel what it is like to be us. We learn that if we speak subjectively – e.g., "I have this desire," "It seems like this to me," "I remember it this way," "In my opinion," etc. – the listener is not triggered to become defensive. If our statement is subjective, it is not "about" the other person "making us feel" a certain way. Nor can the other person argue with our statement. Speaking for Yourself requires being alert to your own subjective world: you can "*see* the images" in your own mind, "*hear* your own inner voice," and "*feel* your own body sensations and emotions." When you are alert and cognizant of your own subjectivity, you can speak about it with responsibility, moment by moment. This is a form of mindfulness that increases the be-attitudes of objective empathy and informed discovery.

Dialogue Therapists in training are encouraged to learn and practice Speaking for Yourself in their own relationships and in conflicts with others. They are sensitized to what a subjective world consists of, and come to see the positive function of lowering emotional threat levels between individuals. When we speak subjectively, we are not claiming objective evidence, as in: "This is the way it is" or "This is the way it happened." Thus, we don't evoke as much defensiveness and argument. Others are more likely to hear what we are saying because they don't have to affirm, agree or endorse the matters objectively.

2   The second component of Real Dialogue is *Listening Mindfully*. Although this form of listening depends on paraphrasing (as do most forms of active listening), it also takes into account the attitude of objective empathy: the capacity to step into another's world and see things from their point of view, to stand in their shoes temporarily. In such a situation, one is able to see, hear, and feel things from the other's perspective. In Listening Mindfully, Dialogue Therapists understand that the emotionally flat parroting of "Here's what I hear you saying" is only the first step into another's world. Listening Mindfully typically begins with "Here's what I am understanding and what I see from what you have just said" or "This is the way it looks to me from what you have said." The listener actually takes a step into the other's point of view or perspective.

At the conclusion of a "unit" of Listening Mindfully, the listener always checks: "Did I get that?" and typically says: "Is there more?" In this way, Listening Mindfully becomes a self-assessment about how well one has heard and stepped into another's point of view, i.e., another's snow globe. For those who practice mindfulness meditation, this form of listening becomes a way of testing your own levels of concentration and equanimity. How clear is your perception of what the other person is trying to convey to you?

The two basic skills of *Speaking for Yourself* and *Listening Mindfully* lead to a shift in attitude for Dialogue Therapists in practice and training. They find that they *remain curious* through their own conflicts and triggering situations much more than they had previously.

3   *Remaining Curious* is the third component of Real Dialogue. What causes us to prematurely shut someone out? Why can't we have conversations with others who have a different point of view? Why do we often automatically feel hurt by a partner who seems to "repeatedly misunderstand" what we are saying? Typically, it is because we listen to the voice in our mind telling us *a story about* what the other person is saying or meaning, instead of listening to what the other person is *actually* saying. The skills of Real Dialogue open up the possibility of listening through difficult emotional states instead of listening only to the voices in our own heads. Often psychoanalysts extol the virtues of "negative capability" and the ability to sit in a state of uncertainty and not-knowing, not longing after facts and reason. This not-knowing leads to new discoveries and creativity because it doesn't prematurely close off the new developments that are surfacing from moment to moment.

When the skill of Remaining Curious is employed, the listener wants to know more and will be able to ask questions to expand the speaker's narrative(s) both more broadly and more deeply. The information and possible details that may emerge from this expansion will enhance the listener's understanding of the other, as well as the emotional baggage and assumptions the speaker brings to the table. Remaining Curious means that partners approach each other with freshness and an "I don't know" mind (the opposite of "I have heard this a thousand times already").

4   *Responsiveness* is a major concern in John Gottman's (1994) research on couples' communication and its effect on their bond. Being alert and responsive to a partner is modeled by the co-therapist team and expected of partners in Dialogue Therapy. Gottman and his colleagues observed many couples for what amounted to thousands of hours. His team found that those couples in which one partner was unresponsive to the other's bids for attention, conversation, or other types of connection, separated or divorced much more frequently than partners who made even "tiny" responses. In DT, there is a built-in structure for developing an interested, engaged attitude toward a partner. Listening partners can exhibit their responsivity verbally or non-verbally. Making eye contact or nodding is a way to stay engaged. Listening partners are encouraged to keep in mind the real concerns and questions the speaker has raised. Also, co-therapists are similarly attentive to each other during the therapy sessions.

5   All of the previously mentioned components of Real Dialogue lead to the capacity for *Witnessing* that shows a partner the reality or fact of having been

seen, heard, and felt, and in that way validated for having expressed a communication. The listener shows they can imagine the world through the speaker's lens and then see that world from the speaker's position and experience. Witnessing does not mean agreeing with, matching, or endorsing the speaker's experience, but *being with it*, respecting and affirming it from the speaker's point of view. For example, the phrases "That makes sense" or "I can see what you mean now" can demonstrate the Witnessing position.

The skills of Real Dialogue are undergirded by the be-attitudes of Dialogue Therapy. When Dialogue Therapists learn and master them, they will be able to carry out all DT methods more confidently and competently. In turn, the be-attitudes and RD undergird all of DT's methods.

Notes

1 For some insightful comments from various actors on their experiences of going in and out of character, the reader may find the award-winning series Inside the Actors Studio illuminating, with descriptions not unlike the discussions of psychodrama contained herein. Those interviews with actors even included a standard set of questions posed to each actor being interviewed.

2 This meditation practice was originally developed by Shinzen Young and is available both on young-eisendrath.com and on unifiedmindulness.com.

★ See Appendix C for the set of Power Point slides for the Introduction to Dialogue Therapy Training.

Bibliography

Banaji, M.R. & Greenwald, A.G. (2016). *Blind Spot: Hidden Biases of Good People*. New York: Bantam Books.

Bion, W. (1959). "Attacks on linking." *International Journal of Psycho-Analysis*, 40, 308–315.

Briñol, P. & DeMaree, K.G. (2012). *Social Metacognition*. New York: Psychology Press.

Flavell, J.H. (1979). "Metacognition and cognitive monitoring: A new area of cognitive – Developmental inquiry." *American Psychologist*, 34(10), 906–911. https://doi.org/10.1037/0003-066X.34.10.906.

Fonagy, P., Gyorgy, G., Jurist, E. & Target, M. (2004). *Affect Regulation, Mentalization, and the Development of the Self*. New York: Other Press.

Freud, S. (1955). *The Interpretation of Dreams: The Complete and Definitive Text* (Strachey, J., Ed. & Trans.). New York: Basic Books.

Gottman, J.M. (1994). *Why Marriages Succeed or Fail . . . And How You Can Make Yours Last*. New York: Simon & Schuster.

Heidegger, M. (1962). *Being and Time* (Macquerrie, J. & Robinson, E., Trans.). New York: Harper Perennial.

Hoffman, D. (2019). *The Case Against Reality: Why Evolution Hid the Truth from Our Eyes*. New York: W.W. Norton & Company, Inc.

Inwood, M. (1999). *A Heidegger Dictionary*. Hoboken, NJ: Blackwell Publishers.

Loftus, E. (1979). *Eyewitness Testimony*. Cambridge, MA: Harvard University Press.

Perel, E. (2006). *Mating in Captivity: Unlocking Erotic Intelligence*. New York: HarperCollins.

Slochower, J. (1996). *Holding and Psychoanalysis: A Relational Perspective*. London: Routledge.

Stern, D.B. (1997). *Unformulated Experience: From Dissociation to Imagination in Psychoanalysis*. Hillsdale, NJ: Analytic Press.

Symington, N. (1993). *Narcissism: A New Theory*. London: Karnac.

Winnicott, D. (1957/1992). *The Child, the Family, and the Outside World*. New York: Perseus Publishing.

Young-Eisendrath, P. (1984). *Hags and Heroes: A Feminist Approach to Jungian Psychotherapy with Couples*. Toronto: Inner City Books.

Young-Eisendrath, P. (2019). *Love Between Equals: Relationship as a Spiritual Path*. Boulder, CO: Shambala.

5 Models (co-therapist and solo), screening, and pragmatics in practicing Dialogue Therapy

Different from other methods of couple therapy, Dialogue Therapy is designed to put the couple center stage from the moment they enter the consulting room. There are always two chairs facing each other where the partners sit, even in the first meeting. Slightly behind those chairs, and outside of each partner's direct vision, are chairs in which the solo therapist or co-therapists will sit (see Figure 5.1). The face-to-face contact of the couple is emphasized, even when there is just one therapist in the room. In this chapter, we give an overview of the two models: co-therapist and solo. In this and later chapters we will also provide the full details of what takes place in each session of each approach.

As long as the method and techniques are used as they have been designed and set out in this book, either approach works according to the principles and theories on which DT and RD were founded. There is no "correct" choice between models. There are, however, many reasons a therapist might elect one model over the other; it may, for instance, be related to their practice set-up and situation (e.g., geography, finances, scheduling constraints, professional community or availability of training). Nevertheless, there are both easier and more choices for interventions (e.g., acting as a Reflecting Team with co-therapists) in the co-therapist set-up.

When you are beginning your practice as a Dialogue Therapist, it is advisable to do so with a co-therapist if possible. While the solo model is very effective, it is best used by Dialogue Therapists who have a degree of mastery of the methods and some experience in making the necessary clinical decisions that are inevitable for the individual needs of each couple as they proceed through the course of treatment.

Co-therapist model

Are two heads better than one? Research tells us little about the advantages of co-therapist models for couples and family work, but our experience tells us this: it is more comfortable for the therapists, and often more comfortable for the couple, too (so they tell us). Having two therapists in the room affords a number of therapeutic opportunities that seem to enrich the therapeutic experience, which may be difficult to operationalize or measure for typical

DOI: 10.4324/9781003200840-5

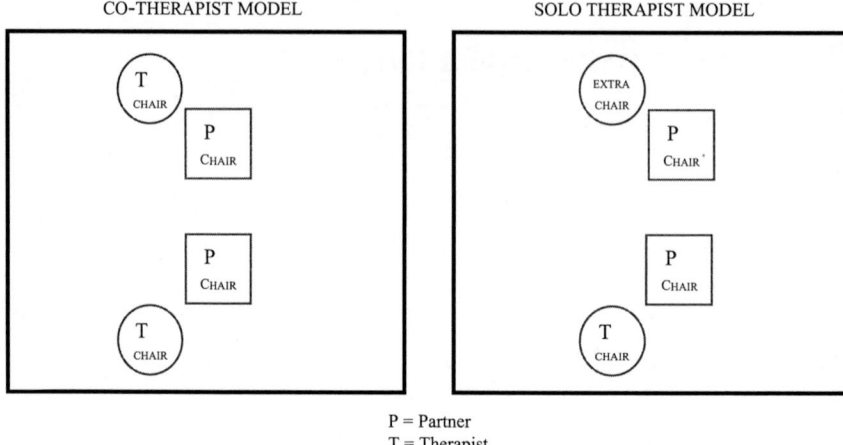

P = Partner
T = Therapist

Figure 5.1 Consultation room setup for two models (furniture is empty)

research. Much more about the co-therapist set-up needs to be studied, but Dialogue Therapy is designed in such a way that therapists benefit from having conversations and reflections together, and typically, the couple benefits from hearing them.

The reasons why a therapist may choose the solo model instead of the co-therapist arrangement are typically more practical than clinical, and include but aren't limited to: costs that the couple pays for two therapists; difficulty scheduling meetings for four adults; a therapist's desire to set a solo fee; or a therapist not having a colleague in their geographical area who knows the method; or even if colleagues are available, an inability to find a good match with a colleague.

Forming a co-therapy team

In forming a co-therapy team, it is important to find a co-therapist with whom you can communicate openly, directly, and clearly, and with whom you can use Real Dialogue during your own conflicts with each other, both in the sessions and in debriefing. Of course, your co-therapist also needs to be certified in Dialogue Therapy or Real Dialogue (if the person is serving as a co-facilitator in RD with you) or to be in the process of getting trained and certified. Even with a certified Dialogue Therapist, though, you must be at ease in communicating openly. If that capacity is not part of the co-therapy relationship, then it is unfair and anti-therapeutic to ask the couple being treated in Dialogue Therapy to be practicing these very skills. As Young- Eisendrath (1984) points out in *Hags and Heroes*:

> [M]easure your own emotional comfort with your potential [co-therapy] partner. If you are anxious, afraid, angry, or submissive during most of your

contacts with the other therapist, you will have the same feelings – and much exaggerated – doing therapy together.

(p. 110)

The felt sense of being a "couple" (a couple of friends, colleagues, or life partners) is often helpful when working with your DT co-therapist. Partnership and sharing, a solid sense of individuation (i.e., one's own autonomy with empathy for another's), and a palpable respect for each other, form the bases of a good working relationship between co-therapy partners. Married or life partners can be ideal as co-therapists when there is not great personal or interpersonal distress in their own lives or relationship.

It is helpful when the co-therapists' styles and notions of practice and technique "fit together." They do not have to be identical, just compatible. It is actually a benefit when the therapists in the co-therapy team are "optimally different." It is a little like the psychophysics notion of "just noticeable difference" – just different enough to challenge, excite, interest, and learn from each other, but not so different so as to provoke high anxiety, avoidance, paralysis, or alarm (Pieniadz, 2014).

We do not feel there is a need to match the individuals in the co-therapy dyad according to gender, age, skin color, etc., or to match that dyad to the partners coming for therapy on these identity dimensions. We encourage therapists to study and address decisions about identity issues, anti-racism, and gender differences in the ways they currently practice. If, for example, you identify as gender non-binary or fluid, do you then advertise and match your client population according to this dimension or not?

Typically, we have found that it works well for a co-therapist team to "mirror the partners" by taking the seats next to their "same sex" individual in the couple, but this kind of mirroring is not a necessity. We encourage the co-therapists to make their own decisions on this matter. When the two therapists identify as the same gender, there is no particular wisdom for choosing the partner (in the client couple) with whom you will Facilitate, Coach or Double (that is, the partner you will be "working with" more). Such considerations require open-ended conversations and dialogue for co-therapists of different skin color or other important identity features.

Matching the therapists' identity aspects to the partners' identity aspects is, and has been, a matter for debate, research, and discussion in the field of psychotherapy as a whole. This matter should be addressed with open-heartedness, open-mindedness, and thoughtful discernment based on the values that one brings to the general practice of psychotherapy. How do you currently make decisions regarding such issues in your own practice? Because DT is a relatively unknown and new model for couple therapy, there may be few Dialogue Therapists available in any community, making it especially hard to match up identity features. However, a degree of planning and consideration on these issues will always be required by both co-therapists (with each other) and solo therapists (with their couples).

The therapists' differentiation from each other, is symbolic of the differentiation we encourage and value between the individual partners in the couple. Appreciation of differentiation is an overarching and thoroughgoing value in this therapy. We try to help minimize assumptions (and projections) based on external attributes, and instead remain interested and curious about the subjectivity of each person as they meet the interactive surfaces of each partner in the couple. Each individual will be supported in speaking for oneself and in listening mindfully.

These considerations notwithstanding, it is important for co-therapists who are very different from each other to have done enough of their own personal therapeutic work, to have worked well with each other in the past, to know something about the different assumptions (e.g., about monogamy, step-families, polyamory, etc.) they are inclined to make about life and love, and to keep these assumptions in a "companionable space" when working together. Such assumptions are bound to undermine our work with couples if they have not been made conscious and explicit to their "owners."

Another note about the Dialogue Therapist's psychology: the emotionally-charged elements of the therapists' psyches (i.e., emotional reactivities that may evoke projections such as parent, child, sibling, etc.) can heavily influence the client couple (Young-Eisendrath, 1984). When therapists' unconscious complexes are emotionally expressed and unexamined or potentially unchecked, they can be harmful to the therapeutic space. The client couple wants to cooperate with the therapists. Clients are in pain and they need help and they need to believe in the therapists' expertise. Unconscious malignant interference coming from unknown or unchecked aspects of a therapist's personality may quickly send the couple running from the therapy. When one therapist recognizes the powerful activation of some kind of emotional complex, it is often best to let the other therapist "lead" the session for a while. The activated therapist can signal this by hanging back, expressing the need for some reflection (e.g., "I just need a minute to think here") or staying quiet and simply listening until the charge has diminished or dissipated.

In the co-therapy model, the sessions (to be described in further detail in Chapter 6) are typically as follows:

Co-therapist model

Session 1: Introduction, Evaluation, Relational History, and Wrap-Up (3 hours)

Session 2: Working on a Conflict, the first session using Real Dialogue (RD) skills, and Wrap-Up (2 hours)

Session 3: Working on a Conflict, Practicing RD Skills, and Wrap-Up (2 hours)

Session 4: Working on a Conflict, Refining RD Skills, and Wrap-Up (2 hours)

Session 5: Role Reversal and Empathy for your Partner, and Wrap-Up (2 hours)

Session 6: Working on a Conflict, Refining RD Skills, and Summary Wrap-Up (2 hours)

Session 7: Six Months Follow-up, and Wrap-Up (2 hours)

Advantages of the co-therapist model include the fact that the total number of therapy *sessions* is fewer than those in the solo therapist model, even though the number of total therapy *hours* might be almost the same. Because there are two therapists, close observation and action (Facilitating, Coaching, Doubling, and other interventions) are distributed between them, but neither therapist should intervene with the other therapist's client, as will become clearer in later chapters. While one therapist is asking a question or making a comment, the other may be closely listening, observing, and taking notes. It is easier to share these tasks in the co-therapist model, and to converse together within the Reflecting Team. Co-therapists also share the emotional burden in holding the tension and anxiety in the room. The anxiety and pressure are more readily contained, perhaps more diffused, with the use of a co-therapy team.

The presence of a co-therapist also allows the ability to check in, check on, and check with each other, as part of caring for the therapeutic frame, process, and the individuals in the room. All co-therapist conversation takes place (co-therapists are seated across from each other in a parallel line with the couple, but behind partners' chairs) with both partners in the room. Partners and therapists face one another at the beginning of each session. (See Figure 5.2). In the Reflecting Team, co-therapists create their own

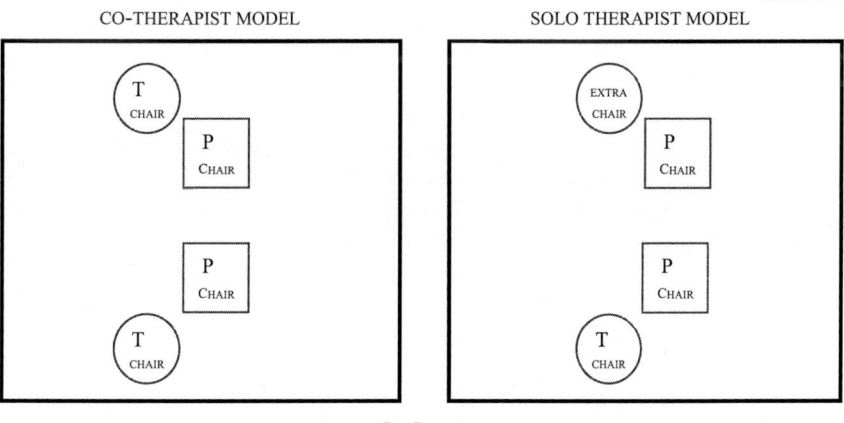

P = Partner
T = Therapist

Figure 5.2 Set-up

dialogue for the couple to hear and witness – a parallel to the partners' voices and dialogue. In hearing from each therapist, the partners also hear how differences can be experienced, shared, navigated, and enjoyed. They witness another "couple" using therapeutic and dialogic skills that they themselves will practice and master. We believe that this kind of "modeling" from the therapists is far more than behavioral; it inspires the couple to see the functions of curiosity and maintaining emotional space as they happen in the therapist couple.

The co-therapy approach also minimizes, but may not eliminate, therapist triangulation, unhealthy alliances, or exclusions as described in earlier chapters. Co-therapist meetings with the couple are at least two hours long and occur monthly during the process of Working on a Conflict.

In this way, the intensity of the sessions is better integrated and the couple is faced with practicing their own skills in Real Dialogue while apart from their therapists. Of course, the month-long wait can be a plus or a minus. It is a plus when partners are less anxious and more self-directed, willing to practice Real Dialogue and consolidate their learning between sessions. It is a minus when one or both partners long for more facilitation of dialogue by the therapists in order to keep them (partners) from losing their way until they feel they have some purchase on the RD skills. Typically, partners become less anxious after their first two co-therapist meetings of Working on a Conflict. They begin to feel the relief of using RD skills the more they practice at home after those first two meetings.

A co-therapist team of Dialogue Therapists offers a strong holding environment for partners' anxieties and often feels comforting to their concerns about a single therapist liking/disliking or preferring one member of the couple. Even the optics of walking into the room with your own "therapist" typically increases each partner's sense of trust. This kind of holding environment is a clear advantage of the co-therapist model (see Figure 5.3).

One of the disadvantages of working in a co-therapy team, however, is the complication of scheduling four busy adults, especially if there is frequent travel required by any of the individuals. Another potential disadvantage is the larger cost per meeting. When there are two therapists (each being paid a fee) meeting for two hours, this can seem like a large financial investment, even though the therapy is time-limited and the number of sessions is limited. Therapists can talk between themselves about how they want to handle payments. These issues intersect with insurance reimbursement requirements, as well. It is possible for each therapist to bill the paired-up "client partner" for each co-therapist session. Since insurance does not typically reimburse two-hour sessions, each client can be reimbursed for only one hour, again making the financial concerns part of the disadvantage of the model.

Another issue with the co-therapy approach involves a more psychodynamic nuance: partners who tend to become socially overwhelmed, who are more introverted or shy, may find that the co-therapist team feels distressing or over-stimulating to the point of it encumbering their learning of the Real Dialogue

5.3a

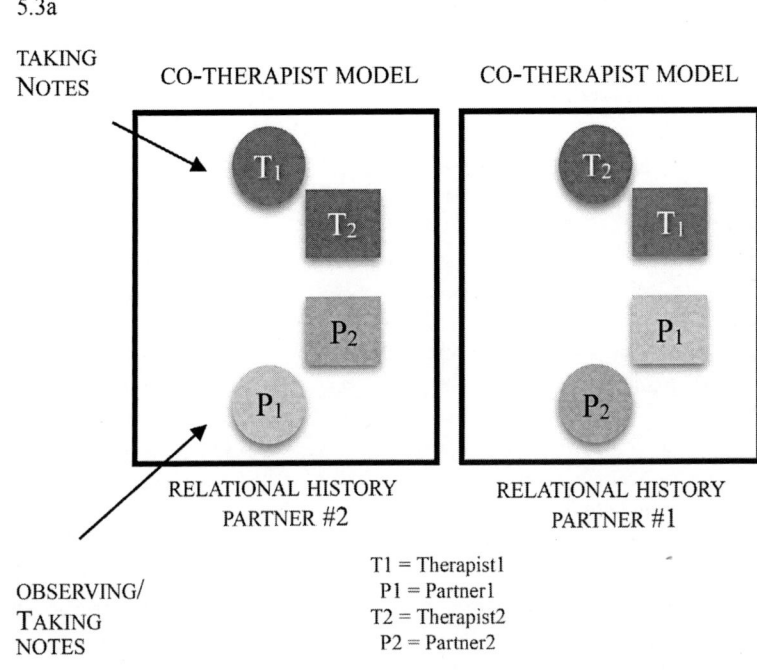

TAKING
NOTES

CO-THERAPIST MODEL   CO-THERAPIST MODEL

RELATIONAL HISTORY   RELATIONAL HISTORY
PARTNER #2   PARTNER #1

OBSERVING/
TAKING
NOTES

T1 = Therapist1
P1 = Partner1
T2 = Therapist2
P2 = Partner2

5.3b

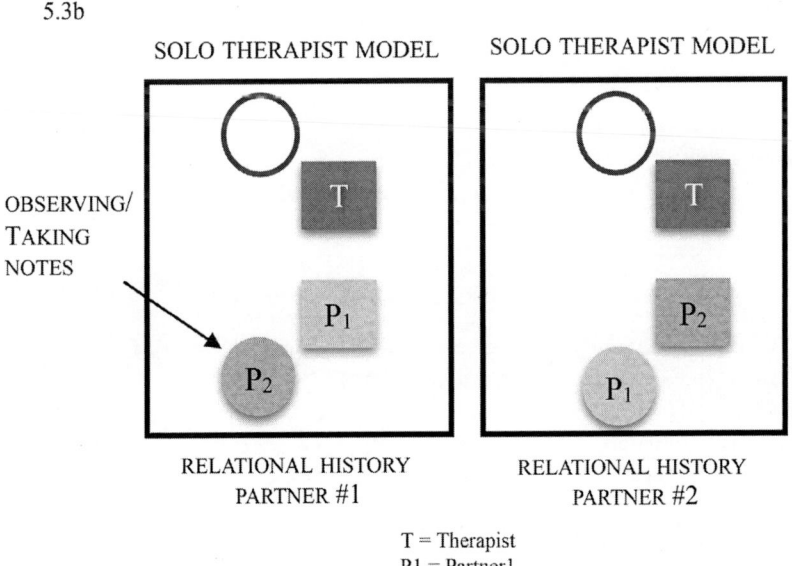

SOLO THERAPIST MODEL   SOLO THERAPIST MODEL

OBSERVING/
TAKING
NOTES

RELATIONAL HISTORY   RELATIONAL HISTORY
PARTNER #1   PARTNER #2

T = Therapist
P1 = Partner1
P2 = Partner2

Figures 5.3a and 5.3b Entering the consulting room

skills, due to self-consciousness. While this can usually be addressed as part of Coaching, Facilitating, Reflecting Team or Unblocking interventions (as described in Chapter 8), some partners may prefer a solo therapist.

In preparation and debriefing, it is important that co-therapists interact with each other both before and after each session. We generally recommend about fifteen minutes on either side of the sessions (for a total of thirty minutes) to discuss ideas, feelings, plans, and assessments. This adds a half hour to the co-therapy approach. While this sounds like an encumbrance, the additional consulting time is typically welcomed by Dialogue Therapists (especially those who are new to the method) because it allows them to process the emotional intensity of the sessions. The solo Dialogue Therapist also benefits greatly from consultation with another Dialogue Therapist when possible. Both co-therapists and solo therapists must consult with other Dialogue Therapists and Real Dialogue specialists in the learning process. The requirements for quick clinical "thinking on one's feet" are demanding in Dialogue Therapy and learning is enriched by consulting with each other. In the co-therapy set-up, the immediate ability to process, in the Reflecting Team, what has just happened and what one is thinking is often very welcome and makes the experience more satisfying and enjoyable for the therapists.

The Institute for Dialogue Therapy, established by Young-Eisendrath some twenty years ago, now offers weekly, online live "Ask Me Anything" (AMA) groups to which Dialogue Therapists (both in training and experienced) can bring their own technical and clinical questions, concerns, and comments for general discussion with an experienced Dialogue Therapy trainer, who facilitates these meetings.

Solo therapist approach

In the solo therapist model, the sessions last sixty minutes (unless paired up into double sessions) and occur at weekly, every other week, or even monthly (after the Working on a Conflict process begins) intervals:

Solo therapist model

Session 1: Evaluation, Introduction, and Wrap-Up (one hour)
Session 2: Relational History of one partner, and Wrap-Up (one hour)
Session 3: Relational History (cont.), and Wrap-Up (one hour)
Session 4: Relational History of other partner, and Wrap-Up (one hour)
Session 5: Optional Continuation of Relational History, and Wrap-Up (one hour)
Session 6: Working on a Conflict, Practicing RD Skills, and Wrap-Up (one hour)
Session 7: Working on a Conflict, Practicing RD Skills, and Wrap-Up (one hour)

Session 8: Working on a Conflict, Honing RD Skills, and Wrap-Up (one hour)
Session 9: Working on a Conflict, Refining RD Skills, and Wrap-Up (one hour)
Session 10: Working on a Conflict, Refining RD Skills, and Wrap-Up (one hour)
Session 11: Role Reversal/Building Empathy, One partner, and Wrap-Up (one hour)
Session 12: Role Reversal/Building Empathy, Other partner, and Wrap-Up (one hour)
Session 13: Refining Skills and Empathy, and Wrap-Up (one hour)
Session 14: Refining Skills and Empathy, and Wrap-Up (one hour)
Session 15: Optional Continuation of DT, and Wrap-Up (one hour)
Session 16: Six-months Follow-Up, and Summary Wrap-Up (one hour)
Session 17: Optional Second Follow-up session, and Wrap-Up (one hour)

One advantage of the solo model is its relative ease in scheduling, making it easier to coordinate the sessions and the process of the therapy. It is easier for the solo therapist to run their own practice and to slot the couple into their regular line-up. The content of the shorter sessions may be easier for the couple to assimilate, and make use of although some couples request two-hour sessions with solo therapists. The emotional intensity of the work and the ways in which insights and skills are integrated in each session may lead to preferring sessions longer than one hour. Partners may feel that they are getting more support in learning Real Dialogue because they come more often. They often begin to practice at home after the second session of Working on a Conflict; hence, they have a longer span of time to develop in RD in the solo process. The important sequence of the Evaluation process (first four or five meetings) demands weekly meetings, if possible. After the Evaluation is finished, then meetings can be more flexibly scheduled according to needs and budgets of the clients.

The financial and insurance requirements for the solo model are easier to handle for both the partners and the therapist. The solo Dialogue Therapist feels more in control of the business aspect and the flow of the sessions than the co-therapists might. And yet, the solo therapist can feel easily overwhelmed by the complex demands of Working on a Conflict, even if the Evaluation process is relatively easy to complete. Once the couple is directly engaged in an enmeshed projective identification, the solo therapist may find the sessions hard to manage and long for a co-therapist.

Some of the typical emotional and management demands for the therapist in the solo model are the following: therapists take all notes for themselves, they formulate all thoughts and interventions, and then (during Working on a Conflict) they must move back and forth from one side-lined chair to the other, acting as their own co-facilitator! At first, this two-chair (one empty chair) set-up may feel unnaturally staged, but becomes more comfortable over time. (See Figure 5.3b.)

One way of easing the solo therapist's job during the Relational History interviews is to record those interviews and then use a computer program to transcribe the recordings (an idea, suggested in a personal communication by Dialogue Therapist, Lisa Lewis, Ph.D.). Because we often refer back to information gathered in the Relational History, it's crucial to have that information in printed form, however it is recorded.

The solo Dialogue Therapist may also face challenges around maintaining the be-attitudes, i.e., an even-handed, open-minded stance toward *both* individuals in the couple. The emotional demands on the solo Dialogue Therapist mean that the solo therapist must adopt good self-care habits (including leaving enough room in the schedule for decompression and rest after a session), participate in the AMA session or another kind of group consultation with other DT or RD professionals, this especially for those who are newly certified, and seek DT clinical consultation with a skilled and experienced DT professional.

Dialogue Therapy is emotionally demanding and challenging, even under ideal circumstances. It is also very rewarding and satisfying because the therapist witnesses the couple's development and growth fairly quickly in the process. This experience will enhance the therapist's skills and mastery in their own relationships with partners and other equals in life. Making use of the mindfulness practices taught in DT training is always very helpful for increasing equanimity and concentration.

Screening

The initial contact with a couple requesting Dialogue Therapy may tell us something about them, but it is little compared to the first actual meeting. Referrals to Dialogue Therapists may come from other clients or professionals (individual and/or couple), from online sources (e.g., a website) or from reading Young-Eisendrath's (1993, 2019) books on couples or from hearing one of us speak publicly, or hearing about DT training.

Sometimes, in the initial email or phone contact, we may obtain some information or "sense" about whether the couple can benefit from Dialogue Therapy, but this matter is only settled through the Evaluation process, which yields a comprehensive Relational History of the couple and each individual. Whether Evaluation occurs in the first three-hour meeting of the co-therapist model, or within four or five hours with a solo therapist, it is comprehensive, impressive to the partners, and conveys major therapeutic effects, whether or not the couple continues into the actual DT process.

Dialogue Therapists should give some thought to the kinds of couples with whom they feel comfortable. They should also have insight into their own capacities for relating – in both couple and other close relationships. Dialogue

Therapists should therefore ask themselves: with what populations would I most like to work (e.g., co-habiting unmarried couples, re-marriages, late-life couples, gay or lesbian couples, blended families, families with adopted children, inter-racial couples, and the like)? Do I have other personal or professional experience with the population of couples with whom I choose to work (e.g., experience in child or adolescence psychotherapy or with co-parenting divorced parents)? Do I know why I have the interests that I do? Am I willing to work outside my comfort zone, say, with a gay couple of a different gender or sex than my own?

Personal prejudices and assumptions that might have gone unexamined (e.g., how you feel about abortion, vaccinations, infidelities, divisions of household labor, religion, money, and so on) can interfere with one's effectiveness as a Dialogue Therapist unless you have worked with your own emotional reactions and can face your emotions with containment and equanimity, at the time they are happening. So it is important not to fall into over-generalizations or category errors or the "*n of 1*" problem in clinical reasoning – viz., "because I have seen one case like this, my experience must confirm that all cases like this are true." It is often an advantage to have had some experience with the issues that partners present, but this is not required (we can and do learn about new experiences in life when we work with them in psychotherapy). Nor do earlier experiences ever exempt us from careful listening and objective empathy for the partners with whom we are sitting.

The pivotal screening for DT takes place in the Evaluation (see template in Appendix A), which is composed of the initial conversation of the couple ("tell us why you are here and what you want" etc.), any Reflecting Team or remarks from the co-therapists or solo therapist about that conversation, the Six Questions, discussion of the Six Questions, and the Relational History interview with each partner, and then the Wrap-Up that gives the concluding impressions from the Evaluation process.

The entire Relational History of a partner always includes a history or account of milestones in the primary relationship, active addictions, violence, infidelity, separation, and the family-of-origin relational history. The Evaluation is so comprehensive and important that Dialogue Therapists may sometimes use a spiral-bound printed version of the Evaluation template (in Appendix A), with the questions printed out and presented in a way that the therapist can easily look up anything needed for supervision, consultation, and briefing before a session. This document can also become the folder for in-session notes for all the sessions, as well as any administrative forms (e.g., insurance and consent forms).

Because the notes from the Evaluation process are extremely important for the therapist to keep in mind to retain the map of projective identification, the notes must be organized by each therapist in a "user friendly way" for that individual. There is no one way that works for everyone. Many therapists like taking the handwritten notes during the Evaluation process and others prefer recording the relational interviews and having notes printed from transcriptions. Note-taking or recording is a major part of the Evaluation process, but not as much a part of the Working on a Conflict or Role Reversal sessions. In those later sessions, therapists can jot down some notes after each meeting or a bit during the meeting. Those notes should be kept with the Evaluation notes. At the time of the six-months follow-up meeting, therapists will want the whole package of notes to recall the patterns and history of the partners.

In general, we recommend delaying or not doing Dialogue Therapy with couples in which substance abuse or addiction or domestic violence is active and *untreated*. Dialogue Therapy is what might be called a "short-term, anxiety-provoking couple therapy," because it can increase both anxiety and aggressive impulses in partners, especially at the beginning of the process. Active addictions and domestic violence should be treated before an individual can be trusted to contain the emotional reactivity generated by DT's sessions. When contraindicating issues are discovered during the Evaluation, Dialogue Therapists will refer the appropriate individuals for treatment while letting them know they can return for DT after being effectively treated.

If a couple is dealing with an active infidelity, Dialogue Therapy is usually effective unless the partner in the affair is not willing to commit, eventually or immediately, to the primary relationship as a monogamous relationship. We state something like this: "If you want to engage in the process of Dialogue Therapy effectively, you will need to give up the outside relationship and be willing to work on repairing trust with your partner. Otherwise, Dialogue Therapy will be a waste of your money and your time, because it depends on commitment to your primary relationship."

In the case of infidelities, the opening one or two Working on a Conflict session(s) are focused on repairing the trust damaged by the affairs. Infidelities have to be addressed at the beginning of the Working on a Conflict process or the trust issues connected will hijack the process, threatening the efficacy of Real Dialogue in regard to other conflicts. Dialogue Therapists use their clinical judgment to adapt the skills of Real Dialogue to inquire into the specifics of partners' experiences of the breaks in trust, keeping in mind the be-attitudes of DT. After the Repairing Trust sessions, the process can move forward.

Dialogue Therapy is not effective for couples who are separating, as a means of settling their differences. However, Real Dialogue for opposing sides can be used to facilitate conversations between separating partners for ongoing co-parenting. Choosing to be in or out of a relationship is a personal choice, not a decision made by the couple, and Dialogue Therapy was designed to work with couples in which both partners are committed to the relationship. If one partner chooses to be out, and the other wants to remain in, there is a great deal of individual work to be done on grief, adaptation, and growth, in life beyond the relationship. Dialogue Therapy is not suited to this work although Real Dialogue for opposing sides might be helpful to a separating couple in which partners have children or a business together.

Individuals with borderline or narcissistic personality organization tend to find Dialogue Therapy's structured set-up, with its demands for constraint, equanimity, and non-reactivity, very difficult to manage. It may be emotionally over-stimulating or could perhaps trigger or evince a sense of abandonment, deprivation, or inadequate mirroring from the therapist. Regardless, when an individual's personality organization is based on splitting the object-world into "all-good" and "all-bad" representations, the therapist can always expect – in any therapy – that the "human objects" in the consulting room will be no exception. Clinical judgment in these cases must be made by the Dialogue Therapist(s). At the very least, these kinds of cases can be managed and handled best within a co-therapist team. We both have worked with couples wherein a partner's borderline or narcissistic psychology is manifest – most often very early on – in the form of "a loved one, hated the other" expressed in one way or another toward the co-therapist(s). Co-therapists need to be alert to such attempts at "splitting" them and converse together about them in the Reflecting Team.

In the solo therapist arrangement, one partner may express their feeling or belief that the therapist is "wrong" and then teams up with the other partner against the therapist. The partner engaged in such splitting may feel persecuted, as though they need to escape a terrorizing or terrifying situation, in which they will never be respected or understood or – much worse – they are annihilated and erased. The solo therapist will need to note this in the Evaluation and decide how to address it and/or if the therapist can manage this partner's reactivity and engage in the process of Working on a Conflict or if the person (or both partners) needs to be referred for individual therapy before coming into Dialogue Therapy.

Another type of observable split is the phenomenon that Pieniadz calls "identity synecdoche" – what cognitive behavioral therapists sometimes call "globalizing" in one's thinking (there are many other terms for this in psychoanalytic literature, too) – whereby a *part* of the person is (mis)taken for their *whole* self. In this situation, a mood or ego-state floods the self to the point of overtaking the person's entire self-concept or identity (e.g., "I feel furious with you, so I am an angry person"). When an individual feels this way, it may be impossible for them to exercise equanimity, curiosity, constraint, containment, and the mindful listening that Dialogue Therapy requires. Their distress is too overwhelming to bracket. And so they cannot stay present with their partner or with the therapist's instructions. These types of splits, exhibited typically by people with personality disorders, can make the Dialogue Therapy process potentially unfeasible. And if they are allowed to continue, then they may undermine, or even destroy, the therapeutic work. And even though a Dialogue Therapist may miss some of these dynamics in the Evaluation, it is imperative that the Dialogue Therapist educate oneself about these personality organizations and be alert to such issues (e.g., see McWilliams, 2011).

Often, the Relational History will give many clues about the personality organizations and attachment styles of the individuals in the couple. Might previous romances be characterized as stormy, impulsive, chaotic? Do the relationship narratives always seem to include all-or-nothing terms rather than, say, more affectively nuanced terms? Other indicators of affect intolerance, rigid projective identifications, or an unstable self-concept may be uncovered in the Evaluation process. Recognition of the difficulties previously described will allow for proper referrals to other helpful resources for such individuals, and may reduce agonizing or feelings for the partners and the therapist(s).

Although Dialogue Therapy sessions are expected to be hard and anxiety-provoking for the clients, the sessions are not intended to engender feelings of being traumatized. When we tell couples that they are good candidates for DT (after Evaluation is complete), we let them know that the process is emotionally challenging and taxing. And even though DT is often taxing for the therapist(s), too, we commit to the whole process when we agree a couple is suitable. At that point, the Evaluation is complete and has invited all of us into our commitment to finishing the process of DT. Once the therapist(s) commits and the partners commit, the intention is to finish the entire process, including the follow-up meeting. In this way, again, Dialogue Therapy is like a theater in which the play opens with the couple center stage and continues through all of its acts until the conclusion (unless the prologue – Evaluation – makes it impossible to do the play).

Money

Dialogue Therapists set their fees based on many conditions (such as, e.g., the marketplace rate for couple therapy), including their own level of expertise (whether they are beginners or masters of the work), which may mean that in the co-therapy approach, couples are paying for two therapists at their hourly fee – often double the rate for a solo therapist. However, the co-therapy approach uses longer sessions and fewer total hours of meeting, as we have made clear. So the financial outlay is larger at the time of service in co-therapy, but more spaced apart (compared to the solo therapist approach), and may require less outlay for the total process than the solo model, depending on a number of factors involving the length of the Evaluation process and the partners' ability to master the skills of RD. In the solo model, the payments are more frequent and smaller at each time of service, spread thinner over time, making it easier for couples to manage the cost and to submit claims for insurance. The solo model, though, may also increase the need for the number of sessions due to the kinds of factors that we previously indicated.

Our experience is that most couples find the Evaluation process compelling and fascinating even though they may balk at first. As they later move through the process of DT, culminating in Role Reversal, typically they complain little about the practical issues of money and commitment. Couples tell us that they learn a great deal in DT, not just about their partners, but about themselves and/or about communication in general, and that over time the effects of this work tend to gain traction and staying power in their lives. Of course, we check back in with our couples at six months after the last session of DT. Though there are exceptions, the majority of our cases have found lasting benefits. Dialogue Therapy is always short-term and time-limited, and so this course of effective treatment actually results in much less expense than many other forms of couple therapy.

Occasionally, Dialogue Therapists set up schedules for Intensive Weekends or Retreats in Dialogue Therapy. These are with an individual couple, not a group of couples. Because DT is a package of sessions and protocols, it can be adapted to intensive formats. The particulars of who/when/why to offer intensives are based on Dialogue Therapists' own professional desires and judgments. Doing Intensives with a co-therapist is very much recommended. The emotional drain is considerable in meeting for two to three hour sessions repeatedly over a limited number of days. These kinds of engagements can be palatable and profitable if co-therapists enjoy working together and feel energized by the challenge of spending intensive time with the couple.

A note about remote/online work and Dialogue Therapy with couples

While it has been very important for psychotherapists and their clients to have the option of working remotely via telehealth platforms or other methods, we have tended to recommend not using such methods for Dialogue Therapy with couples.

However, under the duress of COVID-19 confinement, Dialogue Therapists began to work remotely with couples. The Evaluation process is fairly easy to translate into an online format. The partners sit in their space face to face and the introductory conversation, the Six Questions, and the conversation about the Six Questions are all the same as in the consulting room. When we enter into Working on a Conflict, there is a way to arrange the couple (see illustration in Appendix D) so that a laptop computer is on a table between them. The Dialogue Therapist(s) sees only a profile. The Facilitating, Coaching and Alter-Ego (Doubling) interventions are the same, although they are on a flat screen. It seems that telehealth DT works most easily in the co-therapy model, but solo therapists are doing it with apparently good results.

We, the authors, do not recommend therapist emailing or texting as part of the therapeutic process. While e-mail can be usefully employed to schedule, or re-schedule, or to offer a special agenda (e.g., for those coming for a weekend intensive – see above), it is generally not utilized for other purposes. We have made exceptions on rare occasions by sending a recap or summary of a Wrap-Up to both partners (e.g., when we know we will not be able to see a couple again for a long duration, due to a constraint in their schedule). If more complicated matters arise between sessions, then we ask the couple to wait until we can see them personally. Certainly, if there is a crisis, such as a threat of physical aggression, violence, or suicidality, or a mental health collapse, then we refer people to emergency services. Also, a special "emergency session" of DT can be scheduled.

As we said at the start of this chapter, both models of Dialogue Therapy work well, as long as the structure and process are followed as recommended. Within the confines of the structure and process, many clinical decisions are made instantaneously as the partners, as well as their relationship, come on stage. As therapists become more skilled and familiar with using the methods with a variety of couples, they find that there is plenty of therapeutic creativity within the confines of the method. It is our strong recommendation that beginning DT therapists do not vary the method. And so, we recommend that those interested in using DT or RD become certified and complete the clinical consultation recommended after training, as well as participate in group consultations and discussions about cases until deep familiarity with the method pervades all the therapist's decisions and actions in the consulting room.

Bibliography

McWilliams, N. (2011). *Psychoanalytic Diagnosis: Understanding Personality Structure in the Clinical Process*. New York: The Guilford Press.

Pieniadz, J. (2014, April 13). "Z.P.D. doo-dah: Vygotsky's zone of proximal development and responsiveness in psychoanalysis." *Society for the Exploration of Psychotherapy Integration's (SEPI) 29th Annual Meeting*, Montreal, QUE, CAN.

Young-Eisendrath, P. (1984). *Hags and Heroes: A Feminist Approach to Jungian Psychotherapy with Couples*. Toronto: Inner City Books.

Young-Eisendrath, P. (1993). *You're Not What I Expected: Love After the Romance Has Ended*. New York: William Morrow and Company.

Young-Eisendrath, P. (2019). *Love Between Equals: Relationship as a Spiritual Path*. Boulder, CO: Shambala.

6 Physical set-up and Evaluation in co-therapist and solo models

In this chapter, we describe the set-up of the furniture and "stage directions" for therapists and clients, and give the details of the Evaluation in the co-therapist and solo therapist models of Dialogue Therapy.

Remember that Dialogue Therapy is an intensive, anxiety-provoking, time-limited psychodynamic couple therapy rooted in psychodrama and psycho-analysis. Real Dialogue is the facilitated conversational method embedded in DT. In order for the process of DT to be effective, or to engage with difficult conversations using RD, you must follow the methods, the set-up, and the sessions in the ways they have been designed. The dramatic impact of DT was intended to take place live, in a room, initially with four people – and has been shown now to be effective with only three people – present together or online (if required). There are plenty of opportunities to use your individual clinical wisdom and insight in DT, but they should occur within the structure of the method.

As in improvisational theater, the set-up and containment of the process allow for the freedom to engage with it as individuals.

The physical set-up

One of the distinguishing features of Dialogue Therapy is the physical arrange-ment of the therapy space. From the moment the couple comes into the room, they can see that it is arranged in a very particular way, with four chairs facing each other. The couple's chairs are four to six feet apart, facing each other, and the other two therapist chairs also face each other, though each therapist's chair is slightly behind and to the side of the couple's chairs. The therapists' chairs are set up in such a way so as to be out of the central vision of the person sitting in the "couple seat" (see Figure 6.1).

This arrangement, developed and clinically tested by Young-Eisendrath and Epstein, is most effective for Dialogue Therapy for a number of reasons: it signals to the couple that there is something both dramatic (uniquely staged, as from psychodrama techniques) and ordinary (recognizable, familiar, a face-to-face conversation) about the process to come, and that there is a structure, with forethought, that attends this therapy (Young-Eisendrath, 1984). In the

DOI: 10.4324/9781003200840-6

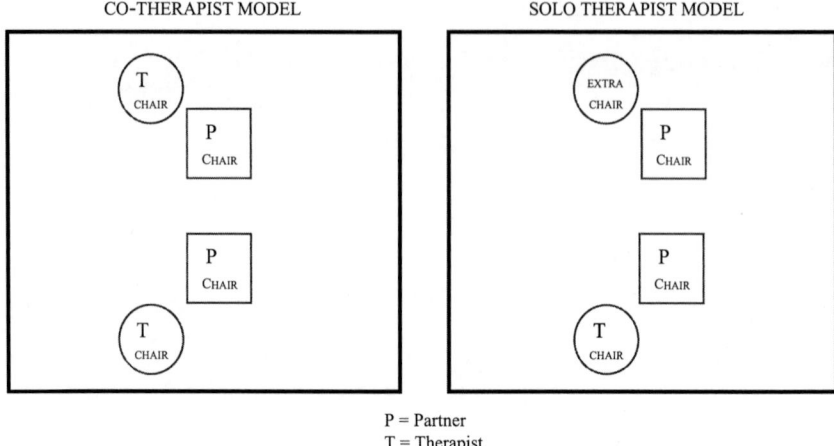

P = Partner
T = Therapist

Figure 6.1 Consultation room setup for two models (furniture is empty)

consultation room, the couple faces each other to talk and are encouraged and supported to do so outside this room, too. The way the couple's chairs are set up is generalizable to the home or other environments outside the sessions, thus facilitating continuity of the DT process beyond the clinical settings. This is a crucial dramatic element in the work: the couple must learn to use their own "steam" and their own idioms, as well as their own personal investment, to improve their relationship. The therapist is not the source of healing in the relationship, a change in the couple relating is.

In the co-therapy model, each partner "has a therapist" and will consult with and be interviewed by that therapist. Thus, the therapist chairs are set up to allow specialized forms of therapeutic support for the client near whom they are seated. Each therapist chair is set up so as to enable leaning forward to coach, prompt, or clarify something for "their" client or to speak as a Double (or Alter-Ego) for the individual when needed. (These latter techniques will be described in greater detail in Chapter 7.) In the solo model, the single therapist moves back and forth between therapist chairs, acting in the coaching, prompting, Alter-Ego or interpreter role for both partners.

The physical set-up may also engender some anxiety in partners in the early stages of the therapy. One of the most common reasons, according to couples, for coming to therapy is that they cannot "face" each other. This set-up, of course, requires their direct eye-to-eye view of each other from the beginning. At the start, their views of each other may seem "stale," as though they "have seen it all and heard it all," but as the Dialogue Therapy progresses there is a freshness in how they see and hear each other.

One of the principles of Real Dialogue, which guides its continued use after the therapy has ended – as a (latent) "sleeper effect" of continued consolidation of new relational patterns post-therapy – is that the couple must learn to be with each other in new ways when the therapists are no longer in their life. This is signaled, at first, by asking individuals to converse with each other, rather than to report to a therapist.

The Evaluation: first session(s)

The first session of Dialogue Therapy, in the co-therapist model, is intended to help the co-therapists and couple to see and talk about the repetitive conflicts (projective identifications) and to clarify some aspects of the problems faced by the couple.

Although the Evaluation serves as an initial screening and history gathering, it is also crucial to the success of Dialogue Therapy and is foundational for the actual dialogue work. This Evaluation is to be understood as a guided and facilitated set of interventions that are "dosed" in a way that allows partners to see, hear, and feel each other more empathically and objectively than they have been doing until that point. The length of the Evaluation session in the co-therapist model is three hours (in one session), and is typically four or five one-hour sessions in the solo model. Often, solo therapists schedule the Evaluation in a cluster of one hour sessions, either with two together, or in a sequence that occurs as close as possible in time.

The Evaluation consists of *four distinct tasks*: (1) a brief explanation of the framework and set-up for the course of the whole therapy, including ground rules, the room set-up, the therapists' roles, and our techniques for working with them, such as Doubling, Coaching, and Reflection (all to be described next); (2) the therapists asking the couple, as partners, to face each other and to engage in a conversation about why they have come for therapy;[1] (3) the Six-Question written exercise intended to allow the therapists to hear from each individual partner, to allow partners to reflect in private about the importance of their relationship, including its benefits and problems, and, to be thoughtful about their partner's response to the same questions (the Six Questions are presented next and in Appendix A). The partners are then guided in disclosing and exploring some or all of their written answers to these questions with the help of the therapist(s) and the structure of the questionnaire.

The last component of the Evaluation is the (4) Relational History of each partner. This is a lengthy history of each partner's view of the relationship; their earlier relationships; and the relational history of their family of origin (see template in Appendix A). This interview is highly structured and follows a logic that is likely to help the therapist perceive quickly the problematic projective identifications between the individuals. At the end of each session, there is always a Wrap-Up.

Here is an example of how we might introduce the work, either before or after we have heard the opening sequence of conversation (at this point, the couple has also already received a printed or digital overview of the DT sessions and its philosophy): "Today, we are meeting in order to do several tasks. We'll conclude by giving you some feedback about your relationship, as well as some information about Dialogue Therapy." The Dialogue Therapists, at this point, also give an overview of the roles they will be taking in the DT process. For example: "As we proceed through this process I will speak with my co-therapist, then we will ask you some questions – we will interview each of you – and also ask that you talk to *each other*. We discourage any cross-talking – or moving outside the designated dialogue space – because that creates disruption and confusion for the way the Evaluation needs to proceed. We will talk with you at the end of the session about our observations, thoughts, and recommendations. Does this all make sense?" (For the solo therapist, the language is adjusted.)

Sample opening dialogue

Before or after the instructions/overview, the therapists greet the couple and sit down in the appropriate chair(s) (see Figure 6.2). Then one therapist says the following: "We would like you to talk with each other about your reasons for being here and what you hope to get from Dialogue Therapy. Please talk only to each other, as if you were having a conversation at home or in the car on the way here. We will observe." (For the solo model, language is adjusted.) The therapists do not interrupt or intervene in any way while the couple is talking, unless there is a hostile or destructive attack that needs to be interrupted. Rather, they look down and take notes, or they look straight ahead at each other; either way, they do not make eye contact with the individuals in the couple. In other words, the therapists occupy a separate space and don't merge with either the couple or one of the partners. Therapists make notes about the content, implied meaning, pattern and rhythms (and other paralinguistic or non-verbal signifiers) of speech, and who speaks when and how (e.g., in what tone, with what characterization of the situation or each other). When possible, they begin to hypothesize the projective identifications to themselves. The therapists also take note of any representations of self and other in each partner's talk; e.g., is there a description, portrayal, or enactment of a puppet-puppeteer, pursuer-pursued, victim-persecutor, or parent-child dynamic in this opening dialogue?

After five to ten minutes, the therapists stop the couple to tell them that they've heard a good sample of how they typically talk together. If there is something obvious to comment on, the therapist(s), e.g., might comment.: "I noticed that you two are especially careful and polite with each other" or "From what I can see so far, what you have said indicates that you are good candidates for Dialogue Therapy" or "There was a lot of attack and defensiveness between you two and we have noted that." Even at this early point, co-therapists may function as a Reflecting Team, the techniques of which are originally described by Andersen (1987, pp. 415–428). The therapist(s) also explain to the couple that observations will be shared in the Wrap-Up and that the session will now proceed to another structured task. It can be comforting or challenging to the clients to hear the therapists speak with each other at this early point in the process.

CO-THERAPIST MODEL

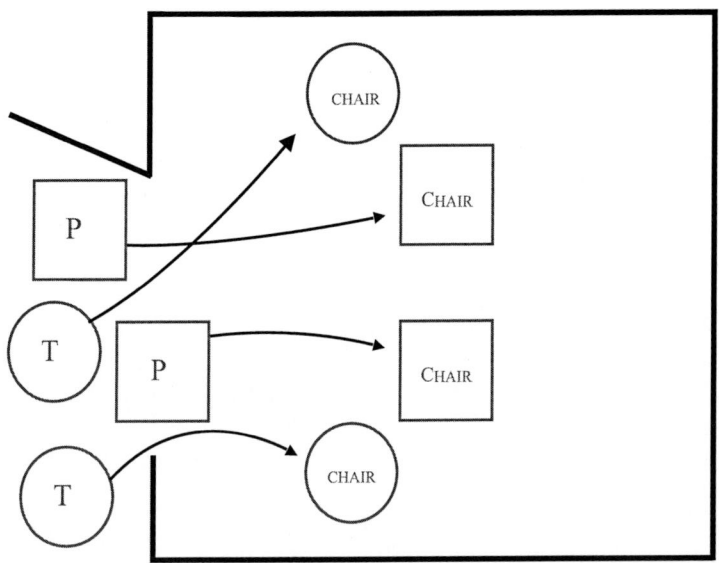

SOLO THERAPIST MODEL

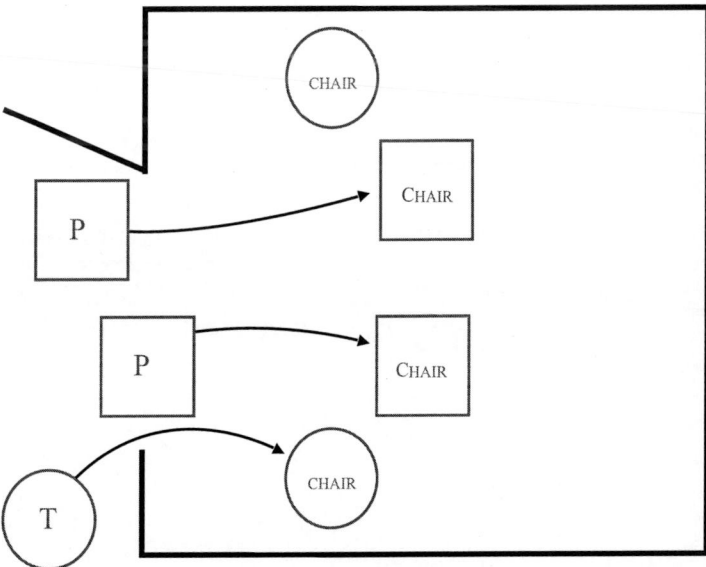

Figure 6.2 Entering the consultation room

The Six Questions

At this juncture, the therapists inform the couple that they will be asked six questions to answer privately in writing on an index card or tablet (provided to them) and that these answers will be shared later with their partner (i.e. they will not be secret). They are told to number each answer, to take their time answering as frankly as possible, and to let the therapist know (usually by looking up) when they have finished writing their answer to each question. Also, partners are told there are no right or wrong answers and that their answers will be used to help the therapists further understand what brings the partners to therapy.

The Six Questions:

1   On a scale of 0–10, rank the importance of this relationship for you personally. How important is this relationship to you? (0 = "I could take it or leave it"; 10 = "It is as necessary as the air I breathe; I couldn't live without it.")

2   What is the greatest problem (or problems) in the relationship, right now, as you see them?

3   What is the greatest satisfaction/benefit (or satisfactions/benefits) in this relationship, for you, right now? What do you value?

4   Write down the number you think your partner gave to the first question. How did your partner rank the importance of this relationship?

5   What do you think your partner said is the most difficult problem (or problems) in your relationship right now? How do you think your partner answered #2?

6   What does your partner think is the greatest satisfaction/benefit (or satisfactions/benefits) in the relationship right now? How do you think your partner answered #3?

After the couple is finished with their answers, the therapists ask to see both partners' written answers. The therapist(s) then confer for a few moments to compare and contrast each individual's responses; they may speak quietly about the things they note, but they don't leave the room, thereby indicating that there will be no secrets in Dialogue Therapy. Solo therapists compare answers on their own and then give the tablets/cards back to each partner before giving further instruction. Solo therapists also may comment briefly on answers or patterns (e.g., "I see from the similarities of your answers that you have spoken together about these things"). Therapists return the tablets/cards to partners before asking them to speak to each other; they return each to their own writers.

Therapists then select one or two answers for which there is a curious or interesting discrepancy or notable similarity – or any other answers or patterns of answering that seem to stand out for the therapists, especially those that indicate anxiety and projective identification – between partners.

The therapists' choice(s) are largely based on clinical experience and intuition, but even therapists newer to this format will find themselves drawn to certain client responses or patterns of response. Often clients are asked to converse about #1 and #3 or #2 and #5. There is no "correct" algorithm for choosing a focus, only that the therapists are helping the couple to begin somewhere, to spark some dialogue, and to come from their private thoughts and feelings to a conversational space between them.

The therapist(s) ask the partners to talk to each other about these responses, trying to make sure that each partner truly understands the other's words. Again, the therapist(s), in their chairs, and off to the side in back of the partners, listen to their conversation: they look and listen for the areas in which there seem to be the most suffering or loss, blankness or deadness, implied or direct hostility, silence or automatic compliance, i.e., the ways of relating that are most emblematic of the couple's complaints. Here, co-therapists may elect to reflect openly together on what they are seeing. Therapist(s) demonstrate Real Dialogue in their own exchanges, especially when they have a conflict about their observations and need to check if they have heard each other accurately, before responding. The Reflecting Team is a clinical and emotional support for therapists and partners. In the solo model, the therapist relies on her own associations and intuitions about what is emerging at this early point and may comment briefly on what has been heard and witnessed.

Although anxieties may run high for partners and therapists at this early stage, it is important that the therapists impart the assurance that they will closely shepherd the process, and that anxiety in and of itself does not forecast a bad outcome in the Evaluation. In all that they say, therapists remind the couple that they (therapists) are not there to "fix their problems," that they are there to respect each partner as having a worthy point of view on what is happening.

In the Reflecting Team, co-therapists may casually convey some educational and developmental information about healthy couple functioning. Therapists find themselves, at various junctures in the process, though most commonly during Wrap-Ups at the end of sessions, in a position to share different kinds of clinical wisdom and suggestions taken from research and other sources, e.g., Gottman & Schwartz-Gottman's (2006, 2015) writings, or Esther Perel's (2006).[2] We consider these psycho-educational teachings to contribute to the couple's "toolbox," to be drawn upon when they want to enhance their insights and skills in their home setting.

The structure of the Six-Question segment is a variation based on techniques that have been used in couples and family therapy for many years: the "unrevealed to revealed differences" exercises – designed especially for facilitating conversations between family members who may feel insecure about speaking when there is conflict (Strodtbeck, 1951; Allen, 1984). By first writing the answers (a private activity), the partner can express oneself while being thoughtful. The therapists provide safety, structure, and moderation after the answers are revealed. The Six Questions act as both an assessment and an intervention device (similar to the function of journaling in weight loss programs). On occasions, of course, one partner "looks to" the other for cues before starting to write, and the therapist indicates that's "against the rules."

Relational History interview

In the final segment of the Evaluation, each therapist (or the solo therapist) interviews each partner separately. The interviewing therapist sits directly across from the interviewee while the other partner sits in the chair behind and to the side of the interviewee. The other therapist sits behind and to the side of the interviewer (see Figure 6.3a).

Those not directly involved in the interview listen quietly, take notes, and are asked not to offer cues, comments, or questions. Naturally, the exception includes requests for repetition (e.g., if something simply wasn't heard). Co-therapists take notes for each other and if there is something the observing therapist is interested in or curious about, and believes will advance the interview, they can also request that the interviewer ask certain questions about that. The co-therapist team may do a bit of reflecting throughout the course of the interview, too, if necessary. And because, with the co-therapy model, the session is three hours long, there is often a five-minute break between interviews.

The observing partner is encouraged to take notes (for their own benefit, to take home) and is provided with a writing tablet for this purpose. When the first interview is completed, the other therapist (in the co-therapy arrangement) becomes the interviewer for the opposite partner, and the first interviewer and interviewee occupy the seats of the previous observers. In the solo-therapist arrangement, the therapist conducts the interviews in one-hour blocks. And the listening-observing partner sits behind their partner during the interview and takes notes (see Figure 6.3b).

A specific template for Evaluation is, as we have mentioned, in Appendix A. Therapists should follow the template as much as possible. Many therapists begin the Relational History with a brief review of the ways partners answer the question, "What are the problems in your relationship?" There may be a need to clarify some of what was said in passing. The therapist takes an interested and engaged tone of inquiry and response with each of the partners, so as to convey to the listening partner an empathic understanding of the speaking partner. The interview covers the following topics:

*   The couple's relationship history, including their foundational story (how and when they met, fell in love, what attracted them to each other, etc.), and when, how, and why the interviewee thought their relationship changed in a notable way (a milestone).
*   Previous cohabiting relationships or marriages, starting with the most recent – and working backward to the first.

6.3a

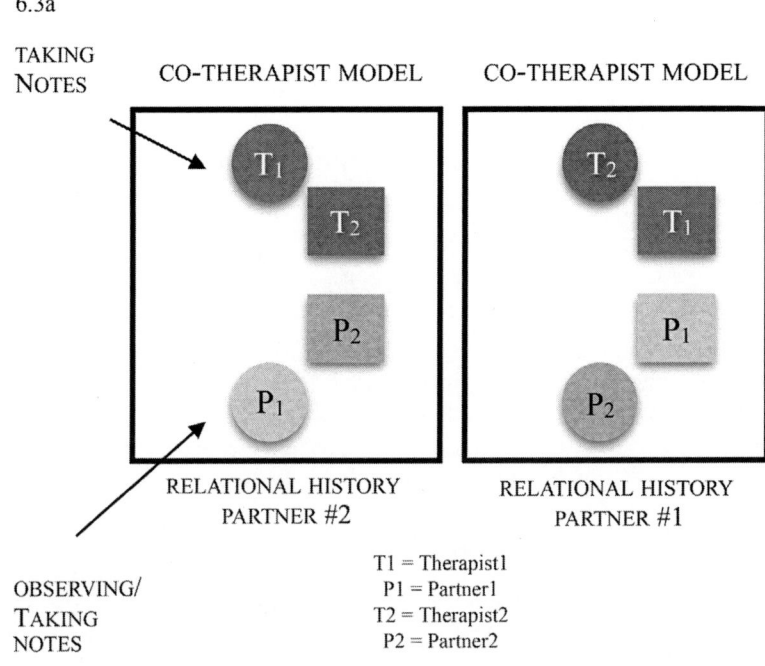

TAKING
NOTES

CO-THERAPIST MODEL   CO-THERAPIST MODEL

RELATIONAL HISTORY
PARTNER #2

RELATIONAL HISTORY
PARTNER #1

OBSERVING/
TAKING
NOTES

T1 = Therapist1
P1 = Partner1
T2 = Therapist2
P2 = Partner2

6.3b

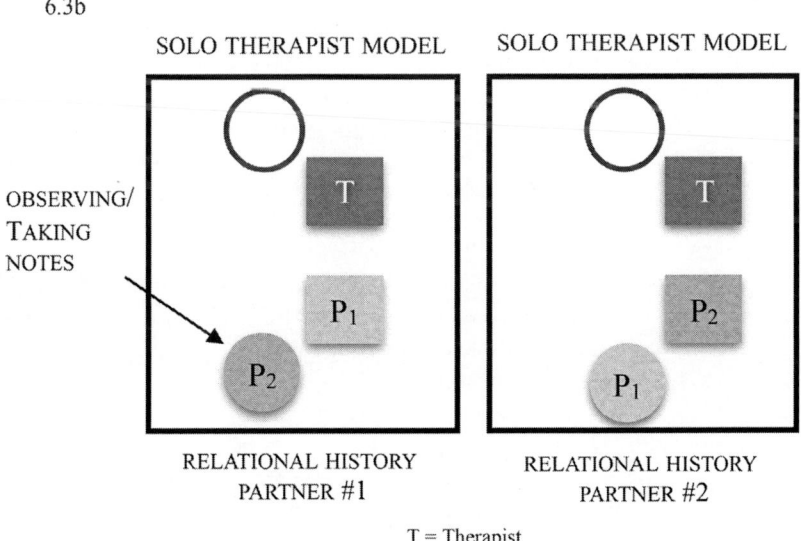

SOLO THERAPIST MODEL   SOLO THERAPIST MODEL

OBSERVING/
TAKING
NOTES

RELATIONAL HISTORY
PARTNER #1

RELATIONAL HISTORY
PARTNER #2

T = Therapist
P1 = Partner1
P2 = Partner2

Figures 6.3a and 6.3b Relational History

- Physical and emotional description, perhaps even "conjuring," of each of the interviewee's parents, specifically from a time before the interviewee entered puberty.
- Relationships with parents and siblings, and some descriptions of family life.
- Brief accounts of grandparents or other parenting figures when relevant.

This segment of the Evaluation session is the longest. Because the solo therapist is both interviewing and taking notes, the interview process is slower than in the co-therapist situation.

The Relational History Interview provides rich information about the partners' identities, life narratives, histories, dreams, conflicts, traumas, and emotional histories. The co-therapists or solo therapist will take note of relationship patterns, themes, and narratives, with an ear for the various projective identifications. The information gained in these extended and detailed interviews scaffolds the work in the actual interventions of Dialogue Therapy.

It is noteworthy that even though the Relational History Interviews are a spotlight on relationships, we often see the individual's unique private life, meaning-making, and associations. Very defining, particular details of a person's life are often observed when an interviewee brings up: (1) a physical injury or illness; (2) other psyche-soma trauma (such as sexual abuse or rape); (3) their particular learning/educational history; (4) special travel experience(s); (5) a traumatic or other extraordinary event in their community (e.g., a murder, or a city block burning down, or perhaps an indelibly unique community celebration); (6) the way something on the world stage, on the scale of 9/11, a tsunami, Hurricane Katrina, the COVID-19 pandemic, changes the way meaning is made; or (7) racial, ethnic, gender, and/or other essential identity cultural shapers of that partner.

Any of these phenomena may have seared itself into the person's psyche, molding their sense of themselves, or the people around them, in ways they feel important to recount in their history. It is important for the therapists to take note of such phenomena and to be able to reference and inquire about them, if they seem to have bearing on the couple's functioning.

In the Relational History, the therapists will sometimes strongly steer the interview because of time limits. It is the job of the Dialogue Therapist to garner a "lay of the land" in terms of relational patterns and idioms, and then make decisions about when and how to re-introduce this material for the couple's consideration, often during Unblocking (to be described in Chapter 8).

Dialogue Therapy's Evaluation sessions are powerful and effective. The Relational History is often noted by partners as one of the "most important" aspects of the overall treatment package. Almost every couple reports, after both partners have been interviewed, that they were extremely moved by listening to their partner's history being taken – even if they "already knew" everything their partner talked about.

They hear this material differently when there is a skilled therapist asking the questions in a curious and empathic way. Partners remark that they never "put together" certain details, sequences of events, or meanings in the ways they heard them in the interview. This experience becomes even more vivid when it's their turn to be interviewed. And these surprises happen despite a certain defensiveness, sometimes felt and expressed by partners entering into DT.

There are, of course, those instances when, whether it is the entire narrative or a small but important feature of the story they have shared, a partner being interviewed reveals something their partner has not heard before (e.g., a death of a sibling). As one can imagine, this can be quite challenging for the partner listening to stay in their seat, continue to be silent, and not interfere.

Wrap-Up

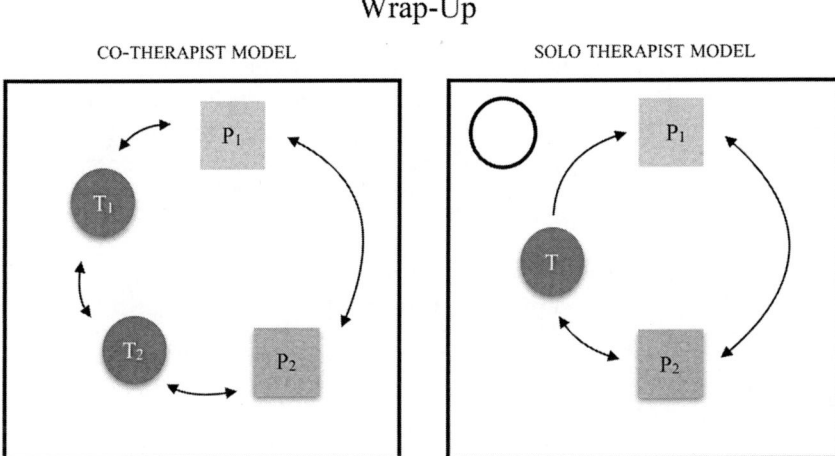

Figure 6.4 Wrap-Up (after the Evaluation)

Wrap-Up (after the Evaluation)

The Wrap-Up in both models serves the purpose of sharing therapists' feedback with clients, and hearing their responses. For this conversation, chairs are moved into a circle (see Figure 6.4).

In the co-therapist model, fifteen to twenty minutes of overview and feedback are given in the Wrap-Up for the Evaluation to the couple through a combination of each therapist's observations and a Reflecting Team interaction between them. Therapists might suggest some readings about important concepts at this time: for example, reading about idealization and projective identification in Young-Eisendrath's (2019) *Love Between Equals: Relationship as a Spiritual Path*. Partners may be asked to read at least Chapter 4 of the book, as it gives more background, theory, and rationale for the Dialogue Therapy work, and explicates the concept of projective identification on which DT rests.

Partners are always asked to review the primers on Real Dialogue, the mini ebooks (available at www.young-eisendrath.com), presented in full in Appendix B. These kinds of "assignments" are based on the therapists' judgments of individual needs of partners and couples. Together, the therapists reflect out loud on their assessment of the couple's interpersonal field, and highlight themes and patterns that emerged during the Evaluation's exercises and interviews. In addition to marking the areas of loss and pain, and the emotional dynamics of the particular projective identifications, therapists also always offer observations regarding the individual and couple's strengths, emphasizing the ways in which they demonstrate commitment to working on their relationship.

In the solo therapist model, the therapist takes about fifteen minutes to do the Wrap-Up and to speak to each partner and answer any remaining questions about the Evaluation. The solo therapist also assigns reading materials and talks about the dynamics of the couple, as previously described. We see this Evaluation as instantiating several of the be-attitudes (set forth in Chapter 4) and the aims of Dialogue Therapy – including informed discovery and objective empathy, remaining curious and expanding the story, mindful Witnessing and constraint, containment and commitment. In this session, we start the partners on a path of speaking for themselves and listening more carefully as well.

Bill and Kathy: samples from Relational History, and Wrap-Up with co-therapists PYE and JP

To help you get a clearer understanding of how the Relational History Interview sounds in an actual case, we are giving a sample next from our demonstration couple Bill and Kathy, whom we mentioned in Chapter 3.

We have permission to use any and all of the recorded materials of Dialogue Therapy with this couple for educational purposes. We also use videos of our work with them in teaching "Foundations of Dialogue Therapy and Real Dialogue" – the basic training course for certification in Dialogue Therapy and Real Dialogue.

Picture the room set-up as in Figure 6.3a.

PYE: *What we're going to do now is: Kathy, you're going to switch chairs and sit behind and to the side of Bill, in the chair I've been in. I will interview Bill. You can take notes on this if you like, or just listen. JP will take notes for me. So, what we'll do right now is go backward in time. We'll start with the present relationship and go backward in time to your earlier relationships: we'll go into your current complaints about the relationship with Kathy, then go back to the beginning of your relationship – to how you fell in love – and the relationship's development. Then, still going backward, we'll go to any other significant previous relationships. We have about an hour to do this. JP and I will keep track of the time. Let's start with something you were implying in the earlier exercise, but maybe not quite willing to say: you might feel, sometimes, unfairly treated.*

BILL: *Yeah, I guess sometimes I feel like . . . I mean . . . I've always had more sort of 9-to-5 jobs, whereas Kathy's more self-employed and has her own schedule.*

And I think I'm a bit envious of that, because I have so much structure. I work in a warehouse, and also deliver around the state as a food distributor. It's pretty physical, driving, loading, or both. I'm waiting for something better.

PYE: *You have a dream of pursuing something else?*

BILL: *Yeah. I'm an artist, a painter. And I do not have time to paint, to have a show in town or something like that. I feel a sort of dichotomy – what I want to do or what I have to do.*

PYE: *Sounds like a struggle there. How, in your mind, or your experience, do those things intersect with your relationship with Kathy?*

BILL: *Well, it feels like more of a personal thing, not so much tied to our relationship. But . . . I guess I think about her having more time than I have. She's also a painter, and she always seems to have more time to paint because of her less structured schedule. So I feel envious of that, maybe a little. Or critical. It's like: I want that, too.*

PYE: *And it's difficult for you to express negative feelings like that to her.*

BILL: *I don't think so. I mean, I'm not really aware of that. Maybe. Yeah.*

The interview with Bill continues with an exploration of the relationship's current and historical functioning and issues. Bill and PYE discuss the "practical and metaphysical" balance the couple seeks in their relationship, and the ways in which these two aspects become polarized at times – Bill embodying the practical (e.g., in his work schedule, which is necessitated by his financial needs), Kathy embodying the metaphysical (e.g., in her artistic pursuits and her attitude that the universe will provide for her even though it is her father who supplements her income). Bill had had an illness in the past several years, too, which is currently being well-managed, and he felt that Kathy had found him "too needy," turning away from him to some extent when he was ill.

PYE: *I'm going to go back to the beginning now. Tell me how you met Kathy, and how and why you fell in love with her.*

BILL: *It was 1996, and we were college students. The first actual conversation we had was when we were walking down this beautiful wooded path to the library. She asked me, point blank: "What do you think of life? What do you think it's about?" And I went into this whole thing I'd been thinking about, that the whole world didn't really exist, and that there was just me, and everything was just a projection of myself. And we totally hit it off.*

PYE: *Like, you were falling in love right away?*

BILL: *Definitely. I was intrigued. Like, this person is really unique. We became friends. We also did a lot of nighttime sneaking around, having fun in the woods. It was a free-for-all campus, with no real authority. I was very shy, though, and nineteen years old. She is four years older than I am. She seemed then like a "grown-up" to me. She was an experienced lady. It was a little intimidating in the beginning. She had actually transferred from another college, and I was fresh out of high school. And I was like, "Whoa! How do I do this?"*

Some aspects of their early relationship are discussed further. But the previous sample gives a foreshadowing of the idealization and splitting, as well as other projective issues, which become clearer as the Evaluation moves along.

Here is the beginning of Kathy's Relational History:

JP: *So, we are going to parallel what PYE did with Bill. I will interview you for about an hour. Let's start with how you see any problems or issues in your relationship right now. Maybe even flesh out some of the things you wrote in the Six Question exercise.*

KATHY: *I feel that both of us have a sort of indecisiveness, a kind of gauziness around some of the decisions we have to make. It makes it hard to move forward in certain areas. In general, we communicate well and have a really good time together.*

JP: *Can you say more about that?*

KATHY: *I don't know. Sometimes I feel like I don't want my reality to bother me. I want things to be exactly how I want them to be, and if they're not, then I'm just kind of grumpy and annoyed about it.*

JP: *What do you think that actually looks like to the other person?*

KATHY: *I think it looks like a lack of engagement and connection.*

JP: *So, you might get quiet or withdrawn with Bill?*

KATHY: *Yeah, I get quiet. It gets hard for me to focus with him. I get disconnected.*

JP: *In what areas does this come up the most?*

KATHY: *Around financial decisions. Or about having children. It's on hold.*

JP: *So things stay fuzzy for longer than you'd like them to, and you want things to be . . . crisper. But when they are crisp, they might not line up with your ideas of how things should go?*

KATHY: *Right. It might end up being upsetting. Like, "I just don't want to deal with this." I pull away. I become curt, less responsive.*

In these brief samples, the reader can see that while the Dialogue Therapists are keeping the overall structure and aims of the Relational History, the therapists do not ask the same questions. They each hew to the structure and intent of the interviews, always keeping in mind the kind of information that will be needed to map the projective identifications, while using their own individual paths to that information.

Clearly, some important information about Bill and Kathy is already emerging. Bill has worries about practical matters, he is concerned about fairness, he harbors envy and criticism toward Kathy's seeming to have more free time than he does (a resource he desires), and he wants more of a balance between work and creativity. Kathy, on the other hand, has a desire for more definition in important areas of their lives, but she knows that this may mean that she does not like the definition in which she participates, which thrusts her into a dysphoric state and distances her from Bill. The Dialogue Therapist then continues with Kathy's version of the couple's foundational story:

JP: *Can you tell me about your experience of you and Bill getting together? What was it like?*

KATHY: *I remember instantly being friends with him and feeling a kinship connection. He was definitely inexperienced, and at the time, I was looking for more of a man. He was incredibly shy. He was not easy to communicate with when it came to being more of a man-woman connection; it was more like we were casual or Platonic friends. Then we started a little company with a third person with whom I had a falling out, and so then there was just the two of us. I was like, "Oh, God." I definitely felt the vibes coming from him, and I didn't know if I wanted to be with him in this way. I began to feel irritation and kind of grumpy, because he was not communicating clearly about it.*

JP: *So, you are implying that if he had been more assertive or direct, then you might've felt a little bit differently about him?*

KATHY: *Yeah, exactly. But then we had our first sexual connection and I was like, "Oh, wait a minute here. I am really responding."*

JP: *Like you surprised yourself?*

KATHY: *Yes. Then I was like, "Ooh, this is not what I thought." So, that was fun. It was great.*

The Relational History with Kathy continues, and aspects of Bill's and Kathy's family histories are also explored.

At the end of the Evaluation Session, both the couple and the Dialogue Therapists turn their chairs to face one another in the Wrap-Up. (See Figure 6.4.)

Excerpts from Wrap-Up with Bill and Kathy (Evaluation)

PYE: *So, basically, we feel you are good candidates for Dialogue Therapy because you have an obviously committed relationship, you have good communication skills, and you both seem to take responsibility for yourself and your own feelings. In that way, you are promising candidates from the outset. To me, there are two or three themes that jump out. One is about making a decision together about whether you want to be parents. We may focus on that in the next meeting. Also, there is a theme about how money plays out in both of your lives. This may be related to the issue of becoming a parent, as well: can you afford what is required financially to become parents? Those are perhaps practical things about which you are being careful with each other.*

It is clear you love each other and that you are good at communicating at an emotionally dynamic level. There are some other things we will return to in our work. One is idealization. You both have your parents elevated into a position where they are amazing, almost mythical [this had come up in another part of the interview]. *So that means you may not feel you can measure up to being adults like them, and here you are, pretty well into adulthood. You might feel that your parents represent the top of the mountain and, "My gosh, we're at the lower part of that mountain." This seems to be an emotional dynamic you share and it may have been one of the reasons you were drawn together: you both have a feeling the world can be amazing, mythical, other-worldly, and so on. With that comes the "possibility of perfection," but perfectionism sometimes takes the form of an inability to make decisions.*

Because, to make a decision means one may have to accept circumstances that aren't perfect – in fact, the world is always mixed, not only amazing. It's both amazing and difficult. In order to make decisions, you almost always have to deal with ambivalence: for example, if we turn left here, we'll miss everything on the right (and vice versa). So, this idealism and perfectionism might prevent you both from feeling like you're "valid" adults, barring you from what adults do: have fun and make income.

JP: *A corollary of this perfectionism, perhaps, is that you both seem to be anxious about a healthy "push" into the adult world – an assertiveness, I guess, that plays out as indecisiveness. It may be a fear of hurting the other person, or a fear of conflict in general. In order to get some closure on certain issues, you may have to mobilize your own "life force": a healthy aggressivity – not to hurt the other person, but to go after something you want. You could each state your own positions and then work your way – negotiate – toward a solution. There is a sensitivity in both of you that is admirable, but which might also keep you from standing up to each other with a certain "life force."*

Perhaps there is also a fear of grief about the things you cannot have after you make a certain decision. The fear of grief can be paralyzing. So can perfectionism. However, there can be a moving forward. But first, you must ask yourself: is it better to have grief that comes from having tried something, despite maybe not having gotten what you wanted, than grief that stems from "the world deciding for you" because you didn't act?

PYE: *Do you have any questions about what we're saying?*

JP: *Or about what has happened so far in this work?*

At this point in the Evaluation Wrap-Up, the therapists make some hypotheses about the functioning of the couple as a unit. In other words, the Wrap-Up example notes things that were in the shared space – the *interactional field* of the couple. In the Wrap-Up, Dialogue Therapists will often also comment on aspects of each partner's family life: for instance, different emotional themes, based on early life experiences in their families, mapping the projective identifications in their relationship, which may have impact on how each partner "sees" or "hears" (or doesn't) the other partner. As Lichtenberg, Lachmann, and Fosshage (2016) write, there may be a "model scene" from childhood, lodged in a partner's mind as an emblem of a defining psychodynamic event for that partner, which they in turn bring to all their relationships, especially their couple relationship (pp. 21–35).

A partner might refer to, or embody, an ongoing pattern of relating between oneself and one's parents or siblings, which may not be easy to verbalize – like music without lyrics – but nevertheless plays a powerful role in the couple's relating through projective identifications. These "other times, other realities," as Modell (1990) refers to them, may present themselves in obvious or subtle ways during the Relational History; and if so, the Dialogue Therapists will incorporate some comments about these different experiences in their Wrap-Up. Thus, the partners' different family backgrounds will result in them interpreting the "same" experience very differently – and the different meanings for each of them can be a great source of misunderstanding and pain. In the Evaluation Wrap-Up, therapists can begin sketching out the reasons, based on their backgrounds, for the partners "missing" or talking past each other when such charged topics come up.

Ideally, the Dialogue Therapist will have at least a rudimentary map of the projective identifications at the end of the Evaluation. If this map can be shared with partners – that is, if the therapist feels capable and confident speaking about it clearly – then it should be shared. If, however, there is a fuzzy sense of it, then the therapist(s) should wait to share it in the Wrap-Up at the end of the first or second session of actual Dialogue Therapy. In Chapter 9, we further clarify how Wrap-Ups sound and are shared with partners. It is in the Wrap-Up that therapists interpret, clarify, instruct, and give an overview of what they see in the relationship and the individuals. During sessions, therapists Coach, Facilitate, and use Alter-Ego and Unblocking techniques with individual partners. Only at the end of the session do they address "the couple" as a unit.

Notes

1 The couple should engage as though the therapists are not there; the therapists are silent while they listen and watch.
2 See also her TED talk "Rethinking infidelity . . . a talk for anyone who has ever loved": www.ted.com/talks/esther_perel_rethinking_infidelity_a_talk_for_anyone_who_has_ever_loved?language=en#t-9335.

Bibliography

Allen, T. (1984). *Personal Communication.*
Andersen, T. (1987). "The reflecting team: Dialogue and meta-dialogue in clinical work." *Family Process*, 26, 415–428.
Gottman, J.M. & Schwartz-Gottman, J. (2006). *10 Lessons to Transform Your Marriage.* New York: Crown Publishers.
Gottman, J.M. & Schwartz-Gottman, J. (2015). *10 Principles for Doing Effective Couple's Therapy.* New York: W.W. Norton & Company.
Lichtenberg, J., Lachmann, F., and Fosshage, J.L. (2016). *Self and Motivational Systems: Toward a Theory of Psychoanalytic Technique* (pp. 21–35). New York: Routledge.
Modell, A. (1990). *Other Times, Other Realities: Toward a Theory of Psychoanalytic Treatment.* Cambridge, MA: Harvard University Press.
Perel, E. (2006). *Mating in Captivity: Unlocking Erotic Intelligence.* New York: HarperCollins.
Strodtbeck, F.L. (1951). "Husband-wife interaction over revealed differences." *American Sociological Review*, 16(4), 468–473.
Young-Eisendrath, P. (1984). *Hags and Heroes: A Feminist Approach to Jungian Psychotherapy with Couples.* Toronto: Inner City Books.
Young-Eisendrath, P. (2019). *Love Between Equals: Relationship as a Spiritual Path.* Boulder, CO: Shambala.

7 Working on a Conflict (WOC) sessions in Dialogue Therapy

What brings couples to therapy? As every couple therapist knows, there tend to be some major categories of conflict that bring couples to a crisis. Not trusting that your partner "gets you" is the number one reason why couples come to Dialogue Therapy these days. This lack of trust may interact with conflicts about parenting and also involve sex, money, division of labor, work/life balance, social life, infidelity, or other difficulties. This list is not exhaustive (only *exhausting* for the couple perhaps) and it certainly does not capture the variations in the ways couples are in conflict or the ways they attempt to cope with it.

Subjectivity and conflict: the snow globe

As most therapists inherently recognize, human subjectivity is complex and conflicted. What is perhaps less known is that our subjectivity is highly individual. At any given moment, what we see, hear, and feel is distinctly idiosyncratic, i.e., subjective, as we are discovering in contemporary cognitive science (see, for example, Hoffman, 2019). When we are emotionally threatened, our psychological defenses intensify and our mid-brains are activated towards the fight-flight-freeze impulse, which is very hard to overcome or side-step. Under these circumstances we are very inaccurate "eye witnesses" and, as Loftus' (1979) research on human memory shows, we cannot be trusted. Even under normal circumstances, we do not "see" the same moon, the same color red, hear the same tone, or feel the same way on a particular mattress – or remember events in the same ways. In times of emotional threat, especially with someone we love and are attached to, we are very likely to defend and protect our own perceptions, insights, and memories.

Although we can do little to change our perceptions and memories, we can strive *to lower the emotional threat level* in order to see, hear, and feel what is going on within our own minds and to begin to explore another's subjectivity. Clarifying perception is one reason why people meditate and practice mindfulness: concentration plus equanimity equals *greater clarity of perception*. Real Dialogue facilitates and teaches partners in Dialogue Therapy the skills of mindfulness under conditions of emotional threat and stress when they are in conflict. The RD skill of *Speaking for Yourself* entails, as we've said earlier, far

DOI: 10.4324/9781003200840-7

more than using I-statements. Of course, it does require using I-statements, but it also requires taking a mental step back and finding a way to speak modestly and subjectively: "Here's how I remember that" or "It's my impression that . . ." or "I don't want to do that because . . ." or "I am sad when you . . ." When we can state something truly subjectively without sneaking in a zinger (e.g., "I feel manipulated by your narcissism"), then it is more likely to be understood by the other person.

A listener cannot argue about our *subjectivity*. We have personal sovereignty over our subjectivity. Our feelings, desires, insights and impressions belong to us exclusively. Each of us inhabits (consciously and unconsciously) our individual experiences. In the skill of Speaking for Yourself, you attempt to speak without trying to control, manipulate, erase, or kidnap someone else's subjectivity. Speaking for Yourself is more than *expressing* needs and desires and experiences; it clarifies that for which you are responsible. Not using "you" or even "we" in making subjective statements (only "I" statements) and staying away from objective claims (such as "This is the way it happened") and rhetoric (such as "Don't you even care about . . .?" or "This always happens because . . .") lowers emotional threat levels. Listeners are better able to hear statements that are not inherently threatening to *their* subjectivity. Confronting, accusing, arguing about facts, and making pronouncements will always elicit defenses and often divert the topic of conversation into a side issue.

Listening Mindfully (i.e., paraphrasing) within Real Dialogue is different from simply paraphrasing, as in "I hear you saying . . ." Listening mindfully requires stepping into the speaker's experience and seeing the world from their perspective. To do this whole-heartedly and freely, you have to recognize that *they too have a world* of subjectivity. By and large, they do not *share a world* of subjectivity *with* you. You have a mind of your own. They have a mind of their own.

In difficult conversations, and all polarizations and polarized negotiations, research shows (see Harvard Negotiation Project, for example),[1] that the overwhelming problems of communication occur in *listening*. According to Dialogue Therapy and Real Dialogue, however, it is also recognized that the first problem may be that the speaker increases the emotional threat level by *faulting* the other person ("You always" or "You never" or "Here's where you fail") or by making claims that are thought to be *objective* ("The fact is" or "The data show") or *rhetorical* ("Isn't it the case that . . ." or "Don't you think that . . ."), as previously mentioned.

Listening Mindfully depends on being able to step temporarily into another's subjectivity and recognize it as a world of its own. This is far more than parroting or tracking a bunch of words. It requires the listener to enter into the other's subjective experience while retaining a grasp of one's own mind. In conflict, especially during projective identification and emotional threat, individuals tend to become entangled in each other's unconscious meanings. Projection of negative thoughts, feelings or traits into the other person is a primary defense of one's own unconsciousness. In place of keeping their ears open, then, listeners talk (self-talk) to themselves about what they want to say to the other person ("Here's why you are wrong about that") or how they feel about the other ("You're an asshole") or how they are going to protect themselves ("I am done, I have had enough"). Instead of listening to the other person, they *listen to the talking in their own minds*. Even with practice and coaching on the skills of Real Dialogue, partners in Dialogue Therapy are often shocked at how little they hear accurately.

Remaining Curious, the third skill of Real Dialogue, requires some ability to Speak for Yourself and Listen Mindfully because these two skills create an intersubjective environment that is more like a *play space* or *dialogical space* in which people can retain a mindful gap. Within that gap, individuals are capable of remaining open-minded, moment by moment. Without that gap, partners and others who are close (or in conflict over opposing sides) believe "I already *know* what you are going to say; I don't have to listen." This is the flavor of projective identification within conflicts. It is the flavor of not being curious. And so, the skill of remaining curious means checking on whether one's eyes and ears are open to something new evolving on a moment by moment basis.

It's really no wonder that we have such a hard time tracking both our own and another's subjectivity. The widely perceived notion that we see and hear "the world out there" and feel "our feelings in here" is a distortion of our actual lived experience. There is no "out there" or "in here," only a jumble of sensations, perceptions, thoughts, desires, and feelings that we remember poorly. Working memory, according to findings in cognitive science, is ninety-nine percent inaccurate, making us ninety-nine percent unconscious most of the time (Solms & Turnbull, 2003).

And so, in the Dialogue Therapy training for clinicians, there is a series of guided meditations on what we're calling the "snow globe of human subjectivity." The snow globe is a metaphor for our individual world of eyes, ears, nose, tongue, body, and mind that seems to be contacting sights, sounds, smells, tastes, sensations, and mental activity moment to moment. We all construct our subjectivity with an "outside" and an "inside." As mentioned, these domains are not clearly sorted because the sights that we "see out there," for example, are mixed with what the mind's eye "sees in here." We may perceive another's neck turning red and thereby feel our own feelings of agitation and conclude: "You are angry at me and I can see it because your neck is red." There are trillions of data points going through our awareness all of the time that are entangled about what's "out there" versus what's "in here." We cannot sort these out. They remain a confusing mixture and always require interpretation. We have our own worlds and have developed language (as imprecise as it is) in order to be able to negotiate and sort out these various "worlds" with the others we care about or depend on.

In Dialogue Therapy training, participants learn how to track their own snow globes of subjectivity. We break down the subjective world into Seeing in/out, Hearing in/out, and Feeling in/out. Because Dialogue Therapists use, Coach, and Facilitate the processes of Speaking for Yourself, Listening Mindfully, and Remaining Curious (as well as Doubling the partners in Real Dialogue), they must begin to learn how to track their own subjective world. What they come to see and understand is how the mix of impressions of the "world" and the "self" are confusing, and how our perceptions of others and our circumstances are inaccurate and limited. In light of this confusion, it is skillful to remain curious and compassionate in our engagements with other subjectivities.

We use the snow globe metaphor because it implies limits of the human world of perception and experience: we are always enclosed in our own perceptions. Through various means – from language to mathematics and science – humans debate and converse about experiences in order to try to establish some kind of consensus so that we can live in the world, in order to retain a degree of congeniality among others. Our experience is always open to debate. When the snow globe is shaken up, as it is in times of conflict, we pay more attention to our own snowstorms (i.e., ways we are swayed by our thoughts and feelings) than we do to the other's subjectivity.

Emotional threat therefore makes it far more difficult to pay attention to another's thoughts, feelings, and experiences, or even to our own, because they get jumbled up as we try to protect ourselves through the defensive habits we learned growing up in a family, especially our well-worn dynamics of projection and projective identification, idealization and splitting.

Most psychotherapists learn to contain and experience their subjectivity while doing therapy, in order to review and decide about when to speak and when not to. Even with general skill or facility in one's consulting room, therapists still find it difficult to have conflicts with family members and loved ones because of the ways that emotional threat is intensified when the stakes are high. Our snow globes of subjectivity make it especially hard to find consensus with those we love. And yet, human beings depend on their attachment bonds with others in order to thrive; when projective identification and emotional threat weaken these bonds, individuals feel unnerved and unmoored. No wonder couples coming to therapy say they cannot "trust" that the partner "gets" them when it comes to some of the most important things they want and need in their relationship. Human subjectivity makes this task of "getting" others very difficult. Emotional threat makes it even harder.

Intersubjectivity and conflict: complexes, projection, and projective identification

Psychological complexes (a term that refers to habituated emotional/perceptual dynamics formed within individual personalities), brought to relationships and interactions with a partner, become especially pronounced through projection and projective identification during times of conflict. At the time of the Working on a Conflict (WOC) sessions, the Dialogue Therapists have already interrogated the foundations of the unique subjectivities of the partners, as well as of the relationship. The therapists should have some ideas of how each person's background comes into play. Each WOC session will reveal details about how each partner's "tribe" and particular relational experiences have a powerful influence during conflicts. When both partners are upset, angry, anxious, or otherwise at the limit of their ability to organize their minds, it can seem impossible to speak or listen.

When Dialogue Therapists begin WOC sessions, they need to take into account the repetitive, destructive, or deadening polarizations underlying partners' conflicts. Typically, projective identification carries the feeling of a life or death situation in which partners feel held hostage. Often, in even the first session of Working on a Conflict, one or both partners feel they will need to leave the relationship if they cannot control the behaviors, thoughts, or feelings of the other person. Normal conflict (without projective identification) can be either threatening or vitalizing; it can enhance a relationship, depending on how it is addressed (Perel, 2006, 2017; Gottman, 1994; Johnson, 2008; Rosenberg, 2015). And yet, the "flavor" of projective identification during conflicts tends to be demoralizing or devitalizing; partners often feel they have "come to the end of their rope" in trying to make decisions or work through even ordinary differences.

In Dialogue Therapy, WOC sessions offer a truly unique opportunity. Partners learn how to manage their emotional arousal and tolerate the state of psychic pain and threat, while also learning how to use the skills of Real Dialogue with a partner they love. Although these conditions may seem to match those in athletic skill development or challenging meditation retreats, they are different from these solo activities because RD is *intersubjective* – not merely subjective. Each partner is sitting face to face with another whom they are asked to see, hear, and feel as a subject like themselves, even while in deep discomfort and reactivity. The therapists help them not only to *stay in the moment*, but to digest the painful moment in such a way that it is felt, metabolized, and relieved. As in the treatment of anxiety, WOC can be compared to what Joseph Wolpe (1958) called "reciprocal inhibition": when a person progresses up and surmounts the anxiety gradient. WOC sessions can be seen even as a type of desensitization because they expose partners to the fears of loss or humiliation while teaching them to encounter their most challenging feelings mindfully.

Pairing the emotional threat of polarization with the experience of being able to tolerate one's own painful thoughts and feelings allows partners to learn incrementally that they have a freedom to work within their own subjectivity and recognize another's. Being able to use Real Dialogue in a personal relationship, during emotional threat and conflict, means partners gain a confidence about working with both themselves and the other person to do "the impossible" – that is, to solve their problems without veering off into attacking or defending themselves when they feel harmed by each other.

The arc of Working on a Conflict in Dialogue Therapy

At the start of Dialogue Therapy, therapists will find that partners often feel lost and agitated in their initial attempts at using the skills of Real Dialogue in WOC and thus require frequent interventions of Coaching, Facilitating, Doubling,

Unblocking or the Reflecting Team (in the co-therapy model). It's important, then, that therapists enter the consulting room well-informed when the WOC sessions begin. In these first two to three hours of the actual DT process, emotional threat levels are typically very high for everyone in the room. Therapists need to read through the notes they have taken from the Evaluation. They need to be clear about partners' histories. They need to hold in mind some kind of picture or narrative or feeling about what the projective identifications are for each of the partners. This kind of scaffolding will allow therapists to hold themselves more confidently in the room. Without it, the impact of the opening sessions of DT can seem discouraging for all parties. But with the review of the couple's patterns and history, the therapist will be able to digest what happens in the session and manage the emotional atmosphere most effectively, so that it is truly *therapeutic* instead of being a war zone of emotional enactments and defeats.

Sometimes, emotional threats (of partners to each other, or one partner to the therapist) seem to overwhelm the therapists' attempts to help individuals see, hear, and feel both their own and their partner's subjectivity. Occasionally, the "music" or emotional tones of a partner's agitation and despair will be felt by the Dialogue Therapist in a way that disrupts or derails the therapist's ability to think and/or pay attention to what is going on. Having a co-therapist is very helpful in these circumstances, as we can then consult, process, cogitate, and interpret what is happening. Without a co-therapist, there can be a sense of total immersion into the couple's dynamics in which the solo therapist fears that going forward with the dialogue process may further harm one or both partners.

When the Real Dialogue process breaks down and the interventions of Coaching, Facilitating, Doubling, or Reflecting Team are not working to help a partner either speak for oneself or listen mindfully, then the therapist needs to engage in Unblocking. In the next chapter, we will go into detail about the nature of Unblocking and how it is used through the DT process. But here, we note that in the early stages (first three or four hours of WOC), a solo therapist (sometimes even co-therapists) may need to override the typical DT process and work with Unblocking with one and then the other partner, even for the whole session. And it looks like this: the therapist moves into the chair across from one partner and asks the other partner to sit behind the first one. Then the therapist interviews the first partner face-to-face (see Figure 7.1).

Typically, the interviewee is the partner who is more agitated or expressing general inability to contain subjective experiences (thoughts, feelings, actions) in order to use the Real Dialogue skills. Unblocking is like a mini-individual therapy meeting. Often, the therapist asks: "What's going on right now?" Or says: "Help me understand what you know about what is going on now." The therapist thereby helps the individual explore the landscape of their subjectivity, but the therapist is also looking for themes of projective identification, which will allow that partner to unlock the defensive posture through which they hear, see, and experience the other partner.

Once unblocked, the person is able to speak or listen in a more skillful way, one that is less triggered and isolated. Through Unblocking, the therapist will

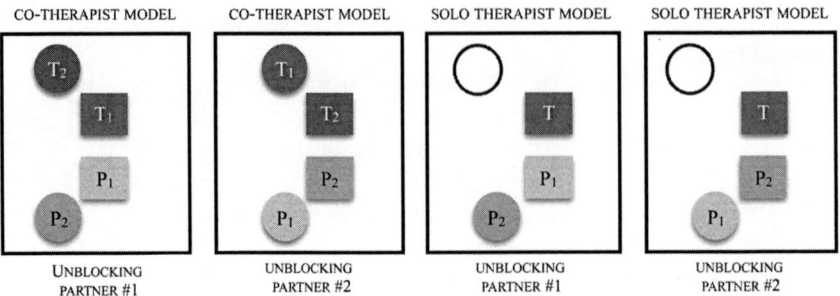

CO-THERAPIST MODEL   CO-THERAPIST MODEL   SOLO THERAPIST MODEL   SOLO THERAPIST MODEL

UNBLOCKING   UNBLOCKING   UNBLOCKING   UNBLOCKING
PARTNER #1   PARTNER #2   PARTNER #1   PARTNER #2

Figure 7.1 Unblocking

establish with the interviewee how to phrase or understand some chunk of experience that is taking place at that moment in the Dialogue Therapy process. Once the therapist and client can agree ("Yes, you got it") on some aspect of the client's experience, then the therapist asks the other partner to return to the seat facing the first partner. The Real Dialogue process can then go forward and the inquiry can continue. Alternatively, the therapist may do an Unblocking interview with the other partner before returning the two partners to facing each other and using the typical DT interventions.

There are some common situations (articulated in the next chapter) in the beginning sessions of WOC in which both partners need the Unblocking process because the level of hostility is high and the humiliation-rage cycle is already underway. Sometimes, Unblocking with each partner is the only process that can happen within the session (especially if it's one hour) because the activation level of threat is too high for the mindful process of Real Dialogue to move forward. In that case, during the Wrap-Up, the therapist(s) reviews why things happened as they did and reminds each partner of the projective identifications and projections that derailed the RD process.

In the course of Dialogue Therapy, however, it's expected that therapists will see the couple gradually become able to contain and experience, as individuals, their own subjective agitations. At the same time, there should be a growing curiosity on the parts of both partners for how they can improve their capacities to explore each other's subjective worlds – using Real Dialogue in sessions and at home – even during the most difficult conversations (e.g., the death of a child) or the most competitive conflicts (e.g., who "works harder" or "deserves more"). In the co-therapist model, by the third WOC (two-hour) session, therapists should witness in each partner some mastery of RD, as well as some capacity to survey thoughts and feelings, even when triggered. In the solo model, the ability of partners to use RD during WOC should improve by the third or fourth hour of WOC sessions. When partners are clearly able to use and understand the skills of RD, during a WOC session, then the DT process can move forward into Role Reversal in the next meeting. In the solo model, it will usually be around the tenth, eleventh, or twelfth hour.

Dialogue Therapists should also notice a perceptible change in their *own* subjective experience at this point: the therapist should begin to look forward to the Dialogue Therapy sessions with partners who are able to use the skills because emotional space, play space, and creativity will naturally enter into partners' dialogue at this point. By the time DT arrives at Role Reversal, there should be greater trust and pleasure in the experience of meeting for all parties involved.

The overall arc of WOC in Dialogue Therapy moves from a sense of over-whelm, dread, or even "this is a disaster" or "this isn't working," to a sense of confidence, trust, and pleasure in partners and therapists. When that arc does not happen in the allotted time in the DT process, then one or more sessions need to be added for developing the necessary skills.

However, the therapist always needs to keep in mind that the skill building requires partners to practice at home, and that the responsibility for the couple belongs to the partners. At bottom, therapists are required to use their clinical skills and judgment in deciding when/how clients move from the WOC sessions to Role Reversal. When partners enter Role Reversal, they should have demonstrated basic skills in using RD while emotionally activated in a WOC session.

Ideals, grieving, and true love

Dialogue Therapists also offer some psycho-education to couples. Sometimes it's offered early on in the therapy. Sometimes, in the Wrap-Up at the end of a WOC session. But we always want couples to know that we empathize with *them* as they traverse the challenging therapeutic terrain of Dialogue Therapy and Real Dialogue. We acknowledge the hard work involved. The skills of Real Dialogue depend on the ability to incorporate mindfulness and insight into one's emotional habits, learned through practice over time. There is a certain type of tension in this exercise of holding or bracketing one's emotional impulses, and it is our impression that many people feel overwhelmed by activation just when it's important to hold oneself. The WOC sessions involve working through the psychic tension and complexity of our emotional lives without splitting ideas, feelings, and relationships into simple "all-good" or "all-bad" fantasies and projections (Klein, 1984; Caper, 2000; Bromberg, 1998, 2006, 2011).

Projection can function to expel either disavowed and devalued aspects of the self or, as seems counterintuitive, an ideal self. The psychology of "splitting" means that the devalued and the ideal are split apart in our sense of self. One way of thinking about the splitting process that includes both ideal and unloved aspects of self is a *morals-based* challenge: one may not want to take responsibility for one's aspirations and competence. If one "owns" their ideal self, then they might feel the moral imperative to "live up to" it, and to recognize its competitive, aggressive, or hubristic elements, and to remain accountable to them. That may be too tall an order for anyone – except, apparently, one's partner!

When the idealized self is projected into the partner, all the criticism one reserves for anyone who falls from a pedestal is visited upon the partner, even as the projector takes the ax to the pedestal, as it were, rendering it unstable. Thinking about this as a therapist, you may recognize that you are uncomfortable if your client praises you too much at the beginning of therapy. The developmental need for splitting can also be understood as a need to keep death and its derivatives as far away as possible from life and *its* relatives because we don't want to experience the vulnerability of our mortality. Again, it is a truly challenging spiritual and psychic task to embrace these seemingly opposing forces of ideal and disavowed. It is not "rocket surgery" (as comedians joke) to understand the challenges for partners to find each other (both self and other) as whole subjectivities, or human beings, as they venture through this psychic jungle of split selves.

Nevertheless, the harder work of holding potential multiple experiences and points of view will be both necessary and more natural as one practices Real Dialogue at home with one's partner. Practice makes . . . easier. Real Dialogue, used during conflict and emotional activation, creates an affirming, yet lighter, hold on mental objects, rather than a defensive, life-or-death clutch, which allows for more fluidity in communication while still retaining boundaries, definition, and thus a relatively stable sense of self. Real Dialogue eventually becomes a gratifying and relieving experience in feeling more whole, integrated, and accepting of reality as imperfect and messy.[2] This work, as many will recognize, is also the work of grieving. It is the work of moving on and growing, making room for what *is* – not staying frozen with what *should* be – and being able to foster true love, not a "dream love."

Freud's "Mourning and Melancholia" (1917/2008) may offer one of the most helpful descriptions of the dynamics involved in the difference between this staying-stuck (melancholia, depression) and moving on (mourning). We see some partners unable to change because they retain an overwhelming attachment to their ideal lover or ideal self and are not able to see the real, sustaining, true love right in front of them.

In WOC sessions, therapists help partners create an emotional space in which they gain compassionate insight into their own childhood wounds as well as compassion for their partner's. Many partners come to Dialogue Therapy saying, "Same fight, different day" (a variation on "Same shit, different day" or "SSDD"). The unconscious dynamics of trying to control, expel, or escape disavowed aspects of oneself, can present many obstacles to hearing, seeing, and feeling another's subjectivity.

Meaning and emotional activation

Within the skills of Real Dialogue, the listening skills (paraphrasing and objective empathy) allow partners to step back from emotional reactivity and concentrate on the content and *meaning* of what the other person is saying. In verifying whether one has listened adequately and understood the other's meaning, one is "tested" on one's concentration by asking "Did I get it?" When a partner says, "That's not exactly what I meant," there may be a moment for developing acceptance or equanimity as one says, "Please help me understand what you meant." When meaning is received and digested by another, we feel more alive and real because we have a sense that we are witnessed, even amidst the chaos and confusion of our own subjectivity.

Everyone's story has the potential to expand in many directions, so it is important for the listener to remain open to hearing more – even if the partner's story does not match the listener's experience. Because of the individual nature of subjectivity, our experiences often diverge considerably. Responding in a validating way ("That makes sense to me" or "I can see what you are talking about") indicates to the partner that one can see things from the partner's point of view, even perhaps while disagreeing with it, and that the partner has a logic and legitimacy. Again, this kind of moment is felt by both people as a relief.

A validating response relies on a temporary suspension or setting aside of one's own point of view in order to allow the partner's subjectivity to have its own truth, its own reality. This is a point where many people become confused: they believe that the validation in this type of response is equivalent to *endorsement*, or *agreement*, or a complete match with their partner's view of things. It is not. To understand and validate does not mean one is in agreement or that the narrative mirrors one's own. It merely recognizes the fact that in every communication between two people, no objective view is possible, as we have explained. Individual reports always include, or emanate from, inherently subjective experience. The aphorism "believing is seeing" is another way we can think about the relationship between interpretation and perception (Gladwell, 2005).

The steps of Real Dialogue trace the ways in which human beings shape, craft, receive, and validate new meanings in their lives. Because of the vast differences between our subjectivities, we need dialogue and debate in order to develop our own meanings and to expand into new views of our existence. As the RD process rolls on, the partner who was the speaker now becomes the listener, and the listener becomes the speaker. The second speaker then has an opportunity to speak and to be listened to in a similar concentrated and matter-of-fact way.

Beginning the session of Working on a Conflict (WOC)

In all WOC sessions, therapists begin by asking the couple – facing each other in the set-up shown in Figure 6.1 – to choose a topic to discuss. This is usually a topic that has some "heat" associated with it, such that whenever the couple raises it at home, they find themselves in a stalemate or in attacks against each other or in an avoidant, shut-down "cold war." Unsolved problems and unmade plans or hurt feelings often become topics for the opening WOC sessions.

At the opening of the WOC session, the Dialogue Therapist asks the couple to "decide together what you want to speak about today, something that is a current conflict." After the topic is chosen, the therapist(s) then say(s) something like the following: "One of you can begin speaking for yourself, then take a break. The other person will then paraphrase what was said. The listener will check on whether the statement was understood before having an opportunity to respond with their own thoughts and feelings. This involves several steps. I/We will help you with this process by using the techniques of Alter-Ego/ Doubling and Coaching." The roles of Coaching, Facilitating, Alter-Ego and Reflecting Team are briefly defined so that partners understand what the therapist is doing in each role.

Coaching and Facilitating Real Dialogue in WOC

Coaching is a method of helping an individual partner improve their ability to formulate their statements in Speaking for Yourself, or to paraphrase in Listening Mindfully. In this role, the Dialogue Therapist will lean in and, in a friendly manner, talk to the partner over their shoulder, as if to indicate: "Let me help you out here." As the individual begins to struggle with the demands of Real Dialogue, the therapist may ask ("What's going on right now?") or suggest ("Think about a way to say what you want to say without a you or we statement") or encourage ("You are doing well here, don't give up"). Facilitating may involve some kind of psycho-educational statement ("Let's keep the threat level here as low as possible") or a suggestion ("Here are some words you can use to begin your statement").

In Coaching or Facilitating, the Dialogue Therapist does not offer interpretations or assessments, but tries to encourage, expand the vision, and help the partner. Typically, the therapist is leaning forward from the chair behind, looking that person in the eye. In telehealth online sessions, the therapist is looking directly at the partner on the screen, and that person is turning their head from facing the other partner, to look at the therapist's screen.

Typically, Coaching or Facilitating is done very frequently in early WOC sessions and is the first intervention offered to an individual when that person has problems using Real Dialogue skills.

Alter-Ego/Doubling

When Coaching and Facilitating seem not to work, then Alter-Ego is the next intervention of choice. Borrowed from psychodrama, Alter-Ego or Doubling involves the Dialogue Therapist crafting a statement for the partner and *speaking it as though the therapist were that individual.* The therapist offers the words tentatively and intuitively, working from their own sense of what the partner is not able to formulate or say, but is implying. When speaking in a session, the therapist always uses the skill of Speaking for Yourself, demonstrating how a subjective statement about desire ("I want this" or "I don't want it"), or feelings ("I am sad because . . ." or "I am excited because . . ."), or opinions ("In my view, it's like this") or memories ("I recall you said . . .") is a powerful, clear, and responsible way to communicate. In the Alter-Ego posture, the therapist is looking down (not into the eyes of the other partner) and is sensing or intuiting into the speaker's subjectivity. The therapist has explained

Doubling and is now working with the partner to find a way to say what the partner wants to say without attacking or blaming or attempting to control the listening partner.

Alter-Ego is a powerful intervention because it is at once intimate and interpretive. It's like homing in on a close-up of the other's psyche. When done well by an experienced Dialogue Therapist, the partner is typically shocked and relieved and grateful. The partner can let the words stand as their own, or they can modify them. Sometimes, the spoken words lead to further Coaching, and then to crafting a statement together to speak back to the other partner.

Therapists also speak in the Doubling role in order to help a partner paraphrase and listen mindfully. The Alter-Ego may offer a paraphrase and then ask the partner to repeat it, or the Alter-Ego may take the Real Dialogue session forward by paraphrasing and asking a question from the perspective of that partner's needs and desires.

Mastering the skills of Alter-Ego increases the Dialogue Therapist's objective empathy and intuition about the particular individual involved. The Alter-Ego/ Double is one of the most important roles a Dialogue Therapist will play; and typically, those in training are reluctant to try it out. The secret to practicing and using this therapeutic technique is to maintain a mindful gap and a sense of humor, while not "trying too hard" to get it "right," because the partner will always help and will always cut the therapist some slack in this role.

The role of Coaching is introduced by saying: "When I am coaching you, I will lean forward and use your name, look at you, and coach you or ask you what is happening – to try and help you to keep finding words." When the therapist introduces the role of Alter-Ego, the therapist says something like this: "When I am speaking as your Alter-Ego/Double, I will speak as though I am you. I will speak this way to help you see how to lower perceived threats and speak for yourself. If you agree that the words express what you are experiencing, then let them stand, and your partner can respond to them as though you were saying them. If you want to change the words, then you're free to do that. We are crafting a statement together."

Emotional relief through Real Dialogue: samples of Doubling and Coaching

While every dialogue is different, here are a few samples from moments of Real Dialogue with some different couples. When the therapist is using Doubling (or Alter-Ego), there is a notation that says **DT *(Doubling)***. Of course, the Doubling is for the person who is named in the line above the aforementioned notation. Check out how the doubling works in these brief examples, in which there is also some *Coaching* and *paraphrasing*:

PAMELA: *Charles, I cannot go on living as we do. Either we have to become more intimate or we have to separate. I am a constant wreck.*
CHARLES: *Intimate? I thought you had given up on sex, I –*

DT (Doubling): *I have a hard time talking about intimacy, and I get very afraid when you say we should separate.*

PAMELA: *Do you really feel that way?*

CHARLES: *Yes. I don't want to lose what we have together.*

PAMELA: *Why can't you say it's me you don't [want to lose] —*

DT (Double): *I want more of a commitment to me personally, not in terms of our children or [our] things.*

Here is another example:

JONATHAN: *The problems begin with what you've done to me [infidelity].*

DT (Double): *I want to know why you weren't faithful to me, why you didn't come to me to talk about your disappointments in our sex life.*

KAREN: *I really didn't think you could take what I had to say. I worried about your self-consciousness and your feelings of disappointment in yourself.*

JONATHAN: *Tell me now.*

KAREN: *I think there's a lot wrong with you —*

DT (Double): *I am uncomfortable taking the lead sexually. I wish you'd take the initiative because —*

KAREN: *Because I wanted to be desired by you. I have a lot of insecurity about my body and appearance, and I've always wondered whether you really found me attractive and —*

And another example:

LARRY: *I want you to quit [the job you complain about all the time] —*

DT (Double): *I want you to take responsibility for what you are feeling. In general, I don't like to hear a lot of complaining, but if you want to get some support or advice, then ask me directly.*

The Dialogue Therapist then asks Larry's partner Louise to paraphrase what Larry's Double has just said:

LOUISE: *You don't want me to complain without having some goal in mind, like getting your advice, right? [Larry nods.] I don't know if I can do that. I get so afraid when I walk through the door. I'm afraid of seeing you and the boys. So instead of dealing directly with you, I usually complain about work.*

Larry is then asked to paraphrase:

LARRY: *You mean you're actually afraid of coming home? Why?*

LOUISE: *Because it seems like I'm the problem around the house. I never get any good —*

DT (Double): *My impression is that no one cares about me, appreciates me. I don't feel at all appreciated for what I contribute to the family.*

LARRY: *That's funny, because I feel the same –*

DT (Double): *I am sorry that you feel so unappreciated because I know how hard you work. Sometimes I feel exactly the same way.*

In these condensed examples, we can see that the Alter-Ego/Double is trying to find words that do not blame, shame, or increase emotional threat, but are subjective and speak for oneself.

Here is another example, a real-time sequence of the therapists' introduction to the tasks in the WOC session. This is the couple Bill and Kathy:

PYE: *Okay, so this is our second meeting after the Evaluation, and we'll be practicing the dialogue skills for which you got a handout in our first meeting. JP and I will be in several different roles here. Sometimes, we will talk to each other about what you've said to us, and sometimes, I'll speak to you like this – I'll lean over and maybe stop you and say: "Talk to me for a moment." Then I might briefly explore some detail with you. Then, I might coach you on how you might proceed in the dialogue. We also have another role.*

JP: *What we would do in this other role is this: let's say Kathy (behind whom I'm sitting) is talking about something with emotional content, and I feel that the emotion or message she wants to convey is obfuscated somehow. I might say, "Let me give it a try." Then I would speak "for" her, as her Alter-Ego or Double, re-wording some of her statements. I will speak directly across to you, Bill – AS HER. Kathy can correct me, if she likes, saying it more the way she would like to say it. She would then be speaking her mind directly to you, Bill, having tweaked what I was saying. Or, she can let what I say stand as is, and Bill you can respond to what her Double just said. PYE will do the same with you, Bill.*

PYE: *Generally speaking, when we are using the Alter-Ego/Double statements, our eyes are down. In that way, we're not looking across directly at the partner, and we will be understood as though we're speaking for the partner nearest us. When we speak as Coaches, we'll directly address the individual nearest us, leaning over toward you, making eye contact, and so on. So, we're teaching or mentoring new dialogue skills. We may give you reminders or prompts about the sequence: e.g., one partner speaking, the other paraphrasing, asking if they got it right, asking if there's more, and validating the speaking partner's position. The roles are then reversed. JP and I will be fairly involved at this stage, whereas in later Dialogue Therapy sessions, we'll be sitting back more often. Dialogue Therapy is a kind of couple therapy that should not depend on the therapist so much. We want you to learn how to use these skills at home, when you're emotionally activated. Right now, we'd like to hear the two of you talk to each other about some conflict you'd like to address.*

BILL: *What do you think? It's probably something about who has decisiveness about money. I sometimes feel that I'm working a lot and you are not and I therefore have less time and energy to pursue the things I want to pursue on my own and with you. That's pretty much the crux of it.*

KATHY: *So, I guess I'll paraphrase. I hear you saying that I put you in a position where you feel like you do too much in a way that isn't working for you. It doesn't support you in pursuing the things that are most important to you.*

PYE [Coaching]: *Let her know if she got the subtleties of what you were saying. You can feel free to add something if you feel she's missed it.*

BILL: *Yeah, I mean . . . I feel it's not something you're doing intentionally or even "doing" at all. It's just sort of how it is right now. I don't want to blame you, but I'm saying I'm working too much in ways that take away from the things I really want to do.*

PYE [Coaching]: *I'm going to ask you to say more about what you are feeling, rather than, "If only we were both working . . ." Tell her that if you feel envious, or angry, or . . .*

BILL: *It sort of comes up in a judgment, when after a long day of work, I have to come home and do something, and I'm like, "Why didn't you do that? You had all day." I think I have expectations for you, because you're not working as much as I am. Then, if you don't fill the expectations, I feel irritated.*

KATHY: *So . . . I hear you saying that when you come home I should at least do some of the things that you don't want to do after working all day, because I have more freedom.*
[Silence.]

JP: *So, one of the things you can do here, Kathy, is ask: "Did I get that?"*
[Kathy asks Bill.]

BILL: *Yeah . . . [Pause.] Hmmm, no, I think there's a little more there. I don't know if I've told you, but I have expectations.*

KATHY: *So . . . you expect me to do things . . . This feels really hard right now. Ok, you feel I have the time to do some of the things you can't get to, but that need to be done, and when they're not done, you feel angry with me.*

PYE [Coaching]: *Kathy could ask you, Bill, what your expectations are . . . or you could tell them?*

BILL: *Alright. But I think this is all tied to the bigger picture of – I just don't wanna be working full time. It often comes down to the dishes (not being done), but it's not really about that. But the fact that I work full time at a job I don't like is what comes up every time I have to cook, and the dishes don't get done.*

PYE [Coaching then *Doubling*]: *Let me try something as your Alter-Ego: I think I would like a policy, which is that if I cook, then you do the dishes.*

KATHY: *So, I guess you were saying . . . you don't know if that would change how you feel about your job . . .*

JP [Coaching/prompting]: *Do you want to . . .*

KATHY: *Oh! Right. Paraphrase. So I hear you saying that if I do the dishes, that would be very supportive to you at this time.*

JP [Coaching]: *And this may be a good place to validate what he's saying, like: "I can see how that would help things in general, and how you would want that, or how that would be helpful to you."*

KATHY: *So I could say that, but I am not going to follow any policy. I mean, I do think of you, but my freedom is the most important thing to me. Which I love.*

Notice how, in the example of Bill and Kathy, what Kathy offered was not a paraphrase of Bill's speaking; she was having difficulty with paraphrasing, finding herself disagreeing with him. This is a juncture at which the therapist might either (1) Coach Kathy on the sequence; that she will get her chance to be the speaker to talk about her view of things, or (2) use Unblocking.

We can also see, in this short example, that a dialogue session may not always follow a clean or direct conversational line. It may take a while before the therapists, and indeed, the partners, can arrive at the main – often hidden or unconscious – points being made. However, it is important for the therapists to intervene to help partners learn and use the skills of Real Dialogue.

It is also noteworthy that what seems *prima facie* to be a "small problem" (the dishes) is really the tip of an iceberg, one that's filled with concerns about envy, injustice, identity, freedom, and responsibility – some of the concerns brought about by ideals of equality and reciprocity. These issues are dressed up in different clothing, and perhaps speak different languages, but they come down to common human needs and desires – including the desire to be understood by another. The need to be understood powers the engine of the WOC sessions and this engine requires the mechanics of Real Dialogue.

It may seem as though these are simple skills, but they are not simple when we are emotionally activated and in a conflict with someone we love (and someone we'd like to control). Witness Kathy's demonstration of difficulty sustaining a mindful stance that would allow her to paraphrase something that sounds straightforward, but that goes against her own grain. All partners and clients in Dialogue Therapy, regardless of their social status or their advantages or their education, struggle with using RD in situations of conflict and emotional threat.

When partners complain about using Real Dialogue

It is worth noting that many partners will complain, saying that using Real Dialogue feels "odd" or "unnatural" or "dumb," or that they find themselves wondering how such seemingly simple interactions can really change anything. At the beginning of the WOC sessions, such complaints are to be expected. But as the therapy moves on, if the complaints continue, therapists wonder if clients are putting up a "resistance" to the method for reasons other than the usual one (e.g., "It's hard to do this when we are emotionally activated"). Resistance is the general psychoanalytic category that accounts for this type of reaction, one that goes against the aims and the thrust of the therapy.

Dialogue Therapists respond in some of the following ways to complaints about the method:

- Real Dialogue *is* odd and unnatural. We remind partners that this is a staged, mindfulness method, and as such, it does not feel like typical conversation. It is akin to practicing scales or rudiments when one is learning the piano or drums, or running drills when one is on an athletic team. In this sense, it *resembles* aspects of the "real" situation in which the skills are to be used, but it is not the same. It is a way to habituate and actually *naturalize* these skills for when they are needed, when one is under pressure, or stress at home.

- Some individuals become almost robotic in their paraphrasing of their partner's words. They may focus on producing verbatim repetition of what their partner just said, looking and sounding like a mechanical doll, or as if they were a mindless, soulless tape-recording of their partner's utterances. When we observe this happening in a WOC session, we stop the listening-paraphrasing partner and either engage in Unblocking or we serve as the Alter-Ego/Double. Partners should be able to feel and appreciate the lively effects of Listening Mindfully compared to, say, parroting – which neither evinces the same feelings nor produces the same enlivening effects.

  When a partner seems to be "just going through the motions" in paraphrasing, that person may be in a state of high anxiety or fear, feeling they have to create a perfect "performance" – so much so that they may have missed the point of remaining curious and interested. It is no wonder, then, that the exercise would feel "dumb" to such listeners – who have, in a sense, rendered themselves dumb. That person has rendered herself dumb – unable to use her own mind to listen actively. This kind of situation may need to be explored through Unblocking.

- Some individuals might not be able to imagine how such "simple" skills – as Real Dialogue – can break up the scar tissue that has built up around the repeated conflicts the couple has had over a long period. Some partners feel that the scars are much bigger and deeper or more petrified than simple "communication skills" can handle, or that these seemingly simple skills are not sophisticated enough for the profoundly complicated psychological problems the couple brings to DT. Again, this may require Unblocking in order for Real Dialogue to go forward.

  Such an attitude of demoralization in the couple or individual often emanates from exhaustion, due to the deadening effect of projective identification. This emotional exhaustion can also manifest as distrust of the therapists or a belief that the therapists are deluded, impoverished, using only puny methods. In such a situation, the therapists may try to "buoy up" or cajole the "depressed" partners about the process. On the other hand, partners may manifest defensive superiority over the therapists and need to win a "therapy competition" to defeat the therapists.

- There may also be a need to feel special in the therapists' eyes: unique, precious, rare. "We've been to many couple therapists, and none of them could do a thing for us." Dialogue Therapists may recognize these as narcissistic defenses in individuals who feel under attack. The attack may evoke feelings of inadequacy in the therapists: e.g., "If only this couple had better therapists, they'd certainly do better."

When the previous scenarios are not addressed *by* the therapists, or handled through Unblocking, the WOC process can be undermined or destroyed. These issues should be addressed head-on as a byproduct of the couple's polarizations and projective identifications.

These days many couples have been exposed to all sorts of self-improvement literature, trainings, and media that extol the virtues of active listening and good communication as the *sine qua non* of healthy relationships. Dialogue Therapists must recognize precisely *how* and *why* Real Dialogue and Dialogue Therapy are unique opportunities for confronting projective identification, maintaining a mindful gap, and learning about subjectivity within a context that explores unconscious meaning within and between partners.

Notes

1 Founded in 1979 at Harvard University, the Harvard Negotiation Project deals in issues of negotiation and conflict resolution. For more information, see: www.pon.harvard.edu/category/research_projects/harvard-negotiation-project/.
2 Cf. Klein's "depressive position."

Bibliography

Bromberg, P.M. (1998). *Standing in the Spaces: Essays in Clinical Process, Trauma, and Dissociation*. Hillsdale, NJ: Analytic Press.

Bromberg, P.M. (2006). *Awakening the Dreamer: Clinical Journeys*. Hillsdale, NJ: Analytic Press.

Bromberg, P.M. (2011). *The Shadow of the Tsunami and Growth of the Relational Mind*. New York: Routledge.

Caper, R. (2000). *Immaterial Facts: Freud's Discovery of Psychic Reality and Klein's Development of His Work*. London: Routledge.

Freud, S. (1917/2008). "Mourning and melancholia." *The Standard Edition of the Complete Psychological Works of Sigmund Freud, Volume XIV (1914–1916): On the History of the Psycho-Analytic Movement, Papers on Metapsychology and Other Works*, pp. 237–258. London: Hogarth Press.

Gladwell, M. (2005). *Blink*. Boston: Little, Brown, and Company.

Gottman, J. (1994). *Why Marriages Succeed or Fail . . . And How You Can Make Yours Last*. New York: Simon & Schuster.

Hoffman, D. (2019). *The Case Against Reality*. New York: W.W. Norton & Company, Inc.

Johnson, S. (2008). *Hold Me Tight: Seven Conversations for a Lifetime of Love*. New York: Little, Brown and Company.

Klein, M. (1984). *Envy and Gratitude and Other Works: 1946–1963*. London: Hogarth Press.

Loftus, E. (1979). *Eyewitness Testimony*. Cambridge, MA: Harvard University Press.

Perel, E. (2006). *Mating in Captivity: Unlocking Erotic Intelligence*. New York: Harper.

Perel, E. (2017). *The State of Affairs: Rethinking Infidelity*. New York: Harper.

Rosenberg, M.B. (2015). *Nonviolent Communication: A Language of Life*. Encinitas, CA: Puddle Dancer Press.

Solms, M. & Turnbull, O. (2003). *The Brain and the Inner World: An Introduction to the Neuroscience of the Subjective Experience*. New York: Routledge.

Wolpe, J. (1958). *Psychotherapy by Reciprocal Inhibition*. Stanford, CA: Stanford University Press.

8 Unblocking

Recognizing, investigating, and addressing projective identification

When partners cannot seem to benefit from the interventions of Coaching, Facilitating, Doubling or the Reflecting Team, then the Dialogue Therapist should use Unblocking – the technique described in this chapter. Unblocking, as we have said, is a kind of mini individual-therapy session with one partner in order to explore and inquire into their emotional experiences and meaning. At these moments of impasse, the therapist, in the solo model, unblocks with the partner who has the most "blockage" (DeKoven Fishbane, Goldman, & Siegel, 2020). In the co-therapy model, co-therapists consult with each other about how and with which partner the intervention should take place. In Unblocking, the therapist moves to sit across from the "blocked" partner to interview him or her and that person's partner sits in the chair behind the partner (see Figure 8.1).

The therapist doing the Unblocking now interviews the client individually (without any help from the partner seated behind) with a particular focus on the block and its attendant associations, feelings, and historical roots. In this moment, the therapist is looking for ways in which the individual is getting snagged on meanings or feelings that unconsciously coalesce around an old parent-child, parent-parent, parent-sibling, or sibling-sibling relation being reflected at that moment in a psychological configuration or dynamic that forms a "complex." These earlier personal experiences often transfer from "another time, another reality," and become projected onto the present partner. These emotional themes require proper identification and a return to their original "temporal space" in order for the individual, the couple, and the therapist to recognize what is happening in the moment.

In Unblocking, the Dialogue Therapist's job is to help an individual partner understand the themes of projection or projective identification for that individual, and to manage or contain their emotional agitation or reactivity in order to return to the Real Dialogue process. Through Unblocking, the reactive partner will begin to open up curiosity about self and partner and thus be able to engage more fully in RD, both in the session at hand and during times of conflict or disagreement at home. In addition, the observing partner can see into, with some objective empathy or even compassion, what has produced this kind of block.

DOI: 10.4324/9781003200840-8

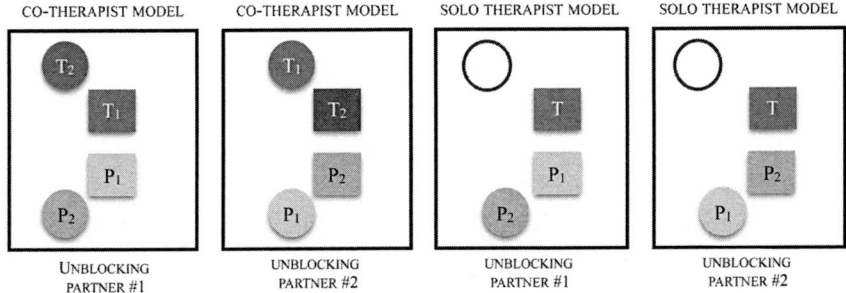

CO-THERAPIST MODEL CO-THERAPIST MODEL SOLO THERAPIST MODEL SOLO THERAPIST MODEL

UNBLOCKING PARTNER #1   UNBLOCKING PARTNER #2   UNBLOCKING PARTNER #1   UNBLOCKING PARTNER #2

Figure 8.1 Unblocking in Co-therapist and Solo models

How does this happen? The process of Unblocking revolves around some of the core principles of psychoanalytic therapy: as a person recognizes that their reaction to a situation in the present belongs to a person, relationship, or situation from an earlier time, which also may not have included a conscious, coherent narrative, or any language at all, they start to untie the knot of these associations. Untying this knot means that they begin to reflect on and see what has happened in their history and their emotional habits, without blame for that situation. Because Unblocking takes place in the heat of the moment of enactment with a beloved partner, the individual often experiences a remarkable *"Ah-ha!"* as does the observing partner. In individual psychotherapy and psychoanalysis, this kind of insight occurs when the therapist does not react or engage with the patient's bids for repetition in an expected way. The patient must mobilize their internal processes to defend against, or, in some way or other, address, cope with, or metabolize the surprise of the "fresh" response of the therapist. In individual psychotherapy, the opportunity for metabolizing split-off material may be resisted or simply passed by. In Dialogue Therapy, however, having been faced with one's partner and with one's unconsciousness, the opportunity for integrating new insights and meanings seems to be enhanced.

"Blocking" can be understood as another term for resisting change because of the threat it poses to the integration of one's "normal" personality or subjective experience. Resistance here can also be understood as a way of holding onto what Pieniadz often refers to as "the package that love originally came in," which does not work for the adults in a mature relationship of love on a two-way street. In Dialogue Therapy's Unblocking process, the blocked partner begins to "decouple" from that old reality and "recouple" with an equal partner in a present-day relationship. It's important to note, however, that in the process of Unblocking, the therapist remains curious and empathic, even cultivating an atmosphere of objective empathy for the earlier players in that individual's life. There is understanding of what happened, but not blame or judgment.

Recognizing a block in Dialogue Therapy

The first step in the Unblocking process is to recognize a block or impasse when it is happening. What signals the therapist that Unblocking should be used? Some indicators of being blocked in the Working on a Conflict sessions include the following:

- The listening partner does not paraphrase accurately, even when repeatedly hearing feedback from the speaking partner that the paraphrase was inaccurate or even after being Coached or Doubled by the therapist.
- The listening partner does not listen at all; instead, the listener continually interrupts their partner, not allowing them to finish their thoughts.
- The listening partner attempts a shallow paraphrase (e.g., "I hear you saying that I hurt your feelings") and then shifts, with a pressured speech, to their own opinions, feelings, ideas, to defend a point.
- The listening partner does not find a way to validate the speaking partner's point of view in any way, or is unable to say anything that resembles the phrase "That makes sense to me."
- The speaking partner does not refrain from "you-statements" or "we-statements," and when they have been repeatedly coached to speak for themselves and given some clues and examples in Coaching and Doubling by the therapist, they continually says things like: "You always . . ." or "You never . . ." or "You were annoyed with me when . . ." or "We can't seem to . . ." or "I feel how you manipulate me . . ."
- The speaking partner is re-telling a well-worn story or running a narrative that seems to involve an adjudication from some outside authority (the therapists, an imagined judge, a parent, or god-substitute); in other words, they are building a case rather than entering a dialogue.

A block is also recognizable in a feeling in the consulting room that this particular moment is suspended in time, in a deadening never-ending loop, a vicious cycle, or a tautological trap. The Dialogue Therapist(s) or the couple may feel exasperated, or desire to blurt out "Enough already!" or, as one frustrated partner put it, they may want to "run, screaming, into traffic."

The therapist(s) may also sense that the couple is in a song-and-dance routine or a habitual "being-nice" that resembles an endurance event, even though the couple may seem to be (temporarily) enthusiastically engaged.

When the therapist(s) recognize a block, they will stop the process by saying something like, "I'm going to stop us here, and we're going to do something else. It is called Unblocking. I'll describe the procedure and the set-up, and then we will change seats."

The Unblocking set-up revisited and some criteria for its use

In Unblocking, the therapist and partner move to the set-up shown in Figure 8.1.

Unblocking is initiated typically with a simple prompt: "What was happening just now?" or "'Do you know what was happening just now?" or "Tell me what you can about what was just happening." Over the course of the Unblocking, the therapist may explore events, feelings, and/or meanings that in other times or in other relationships might seem similar to what just happened in any, some, or all of the following features: (1) emotional tone; (2) "plot," action, or story elements; (3) structure; (4) arrangement of "players" or people involved and their relationships to the blocked partner; and/or (5) result, outcome, bottom line, conclusion.

The interviewer does not typically ask the individual to sort the experiences in this way, but more often explores the meanings and associations the client brings up. The therapist should remain confident that the block is, in fact, meaningful, that it will yield important insights, because sometimes the client is irritated or embarrassed by being "in the hot seat," as it were, subjected to this kind of questioning. Partners can feel "called out" by the therapist. So, the therapist needs to be confident in moving through the interview and not to give into feelings of insult or embarrassment. Unblocking may be a simple discovery process that opens the way to a useful return to Real Dialogue. On the other hand, Unblocking may lead to a deeper inquiry into a partner's emotional history and meaning.

A psychodynamic framework for making use of Unblocking

Often, the process of Unblocking, with the therapist's quick summary or interpretation, allows the partner easily to apprehend the psychodynamic similarities between past and present. The interviewer (therapist) might ask *who* in the interviewee's family of origin may have had strong feelings or reactions to situations parallel to the one with which the interviewee is now struggling. Developmental sequences and stages are kept in mind, also, as the interviewer asks about the age(s) at which certain experiences occurred. Frequency, duration, location, and other details may be explored. Gender, class, and cultural context may also be part of the exploration. Sometimes, there are obvious structural similarities between past and present situations. But most importantly, there are *emotional* or psychological similarities, or what Fonagy and colleagues call "psychic equivalences" between a past situation and a present problematic scenario or impasse (Fonagy, Gyorgy, Jurist, & Target, 2004).

The therapist in the Unblocking conversation may point out the parallels, showing where the partner's reactivity has its basis in something much earlier, e.g., when that person was a powerless child, or perhaps in something more ineffable, something that cannot be verbalized. In conducting such a close, detailed examination of the blocked partner's reactions, the therapist can validate the internal logic, coherence, adaptive design, or integrity that contained the partner's earliest experiences and psychic organizations while helping the partner to see and feel how these reactions do not apply in the current relationship (Slavin & Kriegman, 1992). Relational dynamics in our attachment bonds recur in all of our close encounters with others (Johnson, 2008).

That something old is "being repeated" is sometimes very difficult for partners to believe. Many people have read or heard that psychoanalysis has been "proven to be wrong" or "not working with the facts." Dialogue Therapists need to remain steady in these times and find a clear and simple way to explain how early emotional conditioning becomes habituated. Here lies an opportunity to explain that emotions are often based on "prediction errors" or "confirmation bias": partners can arrive at conclusions that "have more to do with the past than the present" (Dekoven Fishbane, Goldman, & Siegel, 2020). "Showing rather than telling" is the preferred way to proceed as Dialogue Therapists: look for direct relevance and similarities that show how a known emotional experience has been applied in the current moment (Barrett, 2017).

Remind partners to note precisely how projective identification has been operating across time through emotionally charged experiences, from the past, that have been projected onto the current situation. Across the interpersonal space, one person's emotional experience is projected and attributed to the other and, as described earlier, the receiver actually unconsciously *adopts* that projection. When grasped, things make sense to a partner in a new way. In order to reach this point, the therapist(s) may use Unblocking more than once for each partner in the course of a WOC session, but when the partners grasp the paradigm demonstrated through Unblocking, they are often able to self-monitor and unblock themselves without the therapists' assistance.

Sometimes, co-therapists will use a Reflecting Team process to make a decision about a topic for Unblocking. The types of themes, as previously presented, are not exhaustive of all possibilities. Dialogue Therapists use their own clinical skills and intuition to decide on when and exactly what to unblock. Even as we recommend certain criteria and structures, Unblocking is more like a "riddle wrapped in an enigma" than any manual can completely explicate!

When the partners are stopped in their repetitive tracks and these blocks are explored with the therapist, they may uncover "model scenes" in which something crucial, and often pivotal, happened early in the individual's life – scenes which were often emblematic of larger painful patterns in the person's experience of important others (Lachmann & Lichtenberg, 1992; Lichtenberg, Lachmann, & Fosshage, 2016, pp. 21–35). These scenes contain emotional, structural, and relational elements which come forward in a current relationship and are experienced as *identical* to the old situation. The person experiencing the block typically has a "gut feeling" or "feels deeply certain" that the meaning is being attributed correctly in the present relationship. To take responsibility for one's own subjectivity is daunting. People most often feel it would be too much work to *have* the choice to contain reactivity, be reflective, and change course, and see that present meaning is applied "as if" the past is happening again. Our experience shows us, however, that a calm acceptance (usually after some grief work) of personal responsibility is readily available when one understands one's personal history and dynamics and also embraces the relief and joy of being able to be with one's partner without deep distrust and a desire to adjudicate grievances.

Brief examples of psychodynamic meaning discovered in Unblocking

We offer a few examples of blocks that occurred in couples we've seen, illustrating the features aforementioned (emotional tone, "plot" sequence, structure, people involved, conclusions drawn, etc.). These blocks, when manifested in the couples' WOC sessions, were the points at which the therapist(s) stopped the Dialogue Therapy process and used Unblocking to explore the present dynamics.

Emotional Tone: Whenever Barbara – as the speaking partner in the Dialogue Therapy – began to talk about her need for relaxation and alone time, her husband, Charlie, who seemed to be listening intently, would smirk. When he would paraphrase her, each time that he reached the parts about her expressed need for solitary downtime, his nonverbal tone shifted to sarcasm and he raised his hands to put air quotes around these particular terms (something she had not done when she was talking).

In the Unblocking interview with Charlie, he revealed that when he was growing up, if his mother told him she needed a nap, it was really to retreat to her bedroom to drink alcohol. She would emerge a few hours later, drunk, and would not be able to function to arrange dinner, or even make sense. He would feel abandoned, enraged, and betrayed. She had lied to him and spoken in code: "nap," in air quotes, now meant "drink," or "leave you behind," or "become dysfunctional as your caregiver," etc. Now, whenever Barbara wanted time to relax, she reported becoming almost symptomatic with fear that she was doing something wrong, that she would be chastised by Charlie, and she found herself crying all through these so-called rest periods. This latter scenario seemed a clear-cut case of projective identification with Charlie's rejection of her taking relaxation time.

Relaxation was nothing of the sort for Barbara, then; she would experience herself in these moments as a negligent wife and mother, as a sort of layabout, a failure. In the Unblocking interview with Charlie, the connection between his hostility toward Barbara and his anger at his mother for her charades was made obvious. Slowly, he began to see what he was doing with his sarcasm, and he made an attempt to differentiate Barbara's need for solitude from any perceived threat to him or a constitutional flaw in her. She was not abandoning him, betraying him, or losing her ability to function as his partner; she was simply engaging in some self-care, which could potentially enhance her later functioning and feelings of openness toward him.

Action sequence: When it was Samantha's turn to speak, she described her experience of an incident a week before they came to the session: Dianna (her partner) was bathing their toddler daughter and had her back to Sam, over the tub, as Samantha walked into the bathroom. Sam yelled "Heads up!" and then playfully threw a ball for Dianna to catch. Dianna, off guard, started to turn and then slipped, catching herself on a towel bar. She cried: "What the hell?!! You could've hurt somebody! Don't ever do that again!" Their daughter then began to cry and Dianna turned back to the child to soothe her. Samantha walked out, feeling somehow devastated at first, then enraged, and then completely shut down. She had not spoken to Dianna for days now, even though Dianna kept asking Sam what was wrong. Sam remained unresponsive to any attempts to connect. In the WOC session in which Sam told this story, she still could not say what this sequence of actions meant to her, even when Dianna was kind and curious. Sam was dumbstruck, completely blocked.

In the Unblocking interview with Samantha, she described being raised by a single mother. She had a sister four years younger who was severely disabled. She had a few happy early memories of being with her mother and the family dog: at a picnic, on the beach, and so on. She adored her mother and found her sweet, warm, and exciting, and anxious. As it became clearer that her younger sister needed special care, Samantha felt displaced and lonely. She remembered trying to engage her mother in games and activities and calling for her to read to her. Her mother would put her off, saying she needed to attend to Samantha's sister to make sure her sister was safe. The opportunity for connection with her mother would then pass. Feeling bereft, Samantha would try to find various ways to occupy, organize, and amuse herself. To Samantha, everything "always" had to be "on her sister's terms" or based on her sister's needs.

Samantha said that she became quieter, more reserved, a little more anxious, and obsessional as she grew up. She was always looking for possible dangers, things that could go wrong. She wanted to be several steps ahead of Dianna in anticipating what would be needed in any situation, and would become particularly nervous if she thought she would not be able to take care of herself and her family if things didn't go as planned. Dianna had complained that Sam couldn't "let loose and play." A projective identification of Samantha's disowned "preoccupation" (which she had perceived in her mother) seemed to come between her and Dianna.

The sequence that occurred in the bathroom was especially jarring and upsetting for Samantha. She had been relatively relaxed and undefended. She just wanted to play. It was *Dianna* who raised the specter of danger, not her. The therapist helped her connect early sequences with her mother and sister, where Samantha experienced her mother as preoccupied with worry about the little sister, displacing and rejecting Samantha, not empathizing with her feelings while empathizing with someone younger (her daughter in the bathtub evoked her younger sister).

In addition, the Unblocking interview suggested the possible sources of Samantha's long-standing and present anxieties: some anxiety about not being taken care of (she needed care too, not just her sister), some anxiety about the possibility of danger if one dropped their vigilance (most likely an identification with her mother's anxiety), and some doubt about being loved. As this emerged in the Unblocking, and in further WOC sessions, Dianna began to grasp the internal logic of Samantha's anxiety and shutdowns, and showed more patience, as well as more humor, in understanding Samantha's personality.

Structure: In the WOC sessions, when it was Nancy's turn to speak, she would begin talking to Tom about her anger and hurt feelings; he "always seemed to take his parents' side" in the conflicts they had about his parents living with them. Nancy was feeling cramped and wanted to reinstate some privacy in their space, as they used to have. This was one of her deepest desires, she stated.

When it was Tom's turn to paraphrase, he could not refrain from rewording her statements to the point of non-recognition, telling a new story, providing new information or a new defense of his parents. His ability to paraphrase had broken down, and needed Unblocking. In turn, when he became the speaking partner, he had difficulty talking about his own subjectivity. Instead, he talked about the hard lives his parents had, and their values and needs to be close to family. Nancy was not opposed to Tom's parents, and their values or life story; she just wanted Tom to listen to her and empathize and to talk about *his* experiences of his parents living with them. They could not do this.

In the Unblocking, the therapist began to suspect a "structural" issue in the family, i.e., there was a generational boundary being crossed, so that this couple's relationship "envelope" was not being respected or honored by them or by the parents. The Unblocking exploration tested various hypotheses about the reasons for such intergenerational enmeshment. Tom talked about his role in his family of origin, which included being "the fixer" whenever his parents were in distress or challenged by his siblings in their teen years (drugs, criminal behavior, truancy, etc.). He considered his father resourceful, strong, and undaunted by challenges, but also rigid. Tom admired his father greatly and wanted to emulate him. His mother, on the other hand, was fragile; she cried easily when frustrated, and she only seemed happy when "everything was fine."

His father would tend to disappear into his work if he thought his wife was in distress, leaving Tom to be her confidante, comforter, and go-fer. She would often deputize Tom to "get his siblings in line" so she wouldn't have to. His parents told him they were always proud of him, and he felt them to be unerringly supportive of him. He wanted to repay them for all they had done for him by giving them a nice place to live, with good company, when they got old.

In fact, Nancy had fallen in love with Tom partly because of his generosity, and his solid values and ethics about helping others. Of course, the shadow of this aspect of Tom was now falling on Nancy: he was being so "generous" with his parents that it was tantamount to forgetting *her* – except when she was very upset or overwhelmed about something involving his parents. At those moments, Tom felt he was expected to become either "the fixer" again with these "third parties" (his delinquent sibs then, his parents now) or he was meant to disappear into his work, as his admirable father had done. This left Nancy alone to problem-solve, as Tom's mother had been left alone by his father vis-à-vis his siblings.

It took more than Unblocking, requiring some interpretation and gentle suggestions from the therapist, along with continued Coaching, for this couple to come to a mutual understanding and decision that satisfied them both: Tom realized that Nancy *missed* him and their closeness more than she *needed* him (to fix something), that she was actually not going to fall apart when distressed (i.e., she was pretty strong herself), and that his parents would be fine if Tom and Nancy helped them find separate housing nearby. This was a structural solution that had as many emotional and relational blossoms as it had had roots.

Relationships/People Involved: Mason, while listening to his partner Isabel in a WOC session, became increasingly "tensely dead" (to be described next) when he was asked to paraphrase Isabel's statements about her relationship with him after she'd had an affair. (They had come to therapy after the affair was terminated.) The co-therapists had seen in earlier sessions that both Mason and Isabel were extremely articulate and self-aware; they had both been in positive and helpful individual therapy for a long time and were well-versed in the language of self-knowledge. However, in this area, as Isabel spoke of her remorse, her understanding of the reasons for the affair, and her desire for a new closeness with Mason, he began to appear both agitated and over-controlled. When it was time for him to paraphrase her statements, his affect was flat, he seemed suddenly simpleminded or robotic, and all the color left his speech – atypical for what the therapists had experienced of him.

In the Unblocking interview with Mason, he was asked about what he was feeling when he appeared both agitated and dead while Isabel was talking. He said he could only keep "playing possum" until she was done talking, because he could feel himself becoming so enraged and frightened that he was afraid of what would come out. He thought he would hurt Isabel by saying something so violent and devastating to her that she would leave him forever – again for another man.

He talked about growing up with his mother, father, and a brother two years older than him, and said he always knew that his brother "won" his mother and he "won" his father; there was no sharing, no overlap, no negotiation. A positive negotiation, of siblings sharing the parents, is what Juliet Mitchell (2003) calls "The Law of the Mother". His father, who was "his" parent, would exhibit extreme violence toward his mother, calling her names, hitting her, pushing her down – sometimes gravely hurting her – whenever he felt jealous of his own (oldest) son, who seemed to have an enchanted relationship with Mason's mother and never consciously seemed to "get" the connection between this special, exclusive rapture and his father's abuses. The father never assaulted his sons.

When Mason was little, he naturally could not protect his mother; he could only witness the abuse in terror. When he got older, he left home as soon as he could, and was now cut off from his family of origin, with no intention of reconnecting with them.

The therapist in the Unblocking with Mason highlighted the wordlessness of it all. The memories and trauma were so deep in the body that they could not be symbolized. These may be some of the present "as if" experiences, which do not feel "as if" in the moment of occurrence: "There are no words for how I feel when I must compete with another man for a woman I want; I am powerless, I am not an adult man who can contain myself and find a symbol system for communicating my feelings; my body going dead is the only way to survive this onslaught of fear that I will lose her forever and ever" (family cut off = losing Isabel completely). The hurt Mason felt about Isabel choosing another man "over" him was something that was unspeakable. Either he would die or someone else would. Some of these experiences, for Mason, cannot be expressed in words – they are formless, embodied only, and are exhibited as Mason's dissociation when he and Isabel are in the WOC process.

As Mason worked on Unblocking, and in Real Dialogue, and continued his individual therapy, he began to "come back into himself" and to try out different ways of speaking (which Isabel worked hard to paraphrase) about what had seemed an unspeakable storm of thoughts and feelings.

Outcome/Conclusion Drawn: When it was his turn to speak in a WOC session, Josh complained bitterly that whenever he was most vulnerable, his partner, Ellen, would not only withdraw and be unavailable, but she would sometimes even seem cruel and aggressive toward him. While he was saying this, Ellen appeared either deadened, or would interrupt him and tell him he had a habit of exaggerating his pain, or that nothing she could do at those moments would be enough. She had difficulty inhibiting her interruptions of him when it was his turn to speak. He would look stricken, at which point Ellen would throw up her hands and say: "See? It's useless. I'm useless."

The therapist stopped Ellen and Josh, and interviewed Ellen in Unblocking. She relayed a story of her seeing her father crying when she was around four years old, and wanting very badly to comfort him. She went out to the yard and picked some wildflowers, bringing them back to him. She put her hand on his shoulder. He looked up at her coldly, shook her hand away, and said: "What am I gonna do with those? Huh?" He got up and walked away with no other response, no warmth, no gratitude.

She told the therapist: "I decided that day, in my four-year-old self, that I would never, ever do anything like that again. Basically, the four-year-old version of 'It'll be a cold day in hell before I try to comfort some sad guy again.'" Despite their years of being married, Josh had never heard that story. She had been too ashamed to tell it to him. He teared up when she related it (she could not see him, as he was sitting behind her, listening). The Unblocking interview continued with an exploration of the conclusion (the moral of the story, in a way) that she had drawn from her early experience – which was that *she* was inadequate (useless), and any help she could offer in a situation resembling that old experience was forever "useless."

She would not make the slightest effort to comfort her male partner, lest she be shamed, rejected, and rendered helpless, unimportant, and unworthy again.

This pattern had been so petrified in her that she was beginning to exhibit it with their young son. In the WOC session, Ellen began to see that she was very important to Josh, that she affected him deeply, and that her attempts to comfort him would not only be welcomed but appreciated, absorbed. Josh, who had been locked into a projective identification with Ellen, ashamed of his own vulnerability and need, and going in and out of deciding whether he would not let her in anymore, became more relaxed and open about sharing his more vulnerable side. Ellen gradually, and awkwardly, made more attempts to soothe him at these moments.

Cultural/racial/gender wounds: Remember Devan and Kendal from Chapter 3? Devan is an African American Jehovah's Witness who takes her religion to heart. She is active in the church community and believes that everything good within her has been strengthened by becoming a Witness, which she became just five years ago. She is thirty-five years old and has one child with Kendal. Kendal, thirty-six, is Rastafarian, although he doesn't feel it's exactly his religion but more his "lifestyle." Kendal is White.

In their first WOC, Kendal seemed unable to paraphrase what Devan said about the "most meaningful part of life is my relationship to God. God is personal and divine, to me. That's why I feel completely enraged that you call my religion a 'cult' or you make fun of it. I don't get it. I don't know how you could love me and not respect my religion." At first, the therapist coached Kendal on what Devan was saying, especially the gist of making fun of what was of greatest value to her. Each time the therapist tried to get Kendal to paraphrase, he missed the part about "making fun" of her religion. Finally, the therapist switched seats and began to interview Kendal in Unblocking.

Kendal said that he often felt ashamed of the fact that he couldn't believe in Devan's religion. He feared that it was a deficit or defect in him. He was afraid that it might be related to some "hidden racism" from his early years when his parents, poor farmers in northern Vermont (originally from Quebec), were apprehensive about relating to Mexican immigrants (who came up to work on the harvest). His parents would say "these people are weird and have some weird beliefs."

At the same time, his grandparents, being Francophones, did not speak English and Kendal often felt *they* were "weird," but he pretended to love them nonetheless. Spending summers at his grandparents' farm near Quebec City, Kendal felt isolated and left out. He couldn't speak their language and he often felt that he was disliked by his cousins. He spent a lot of time alone in the summers, even though he worked on the farm. His grandparents were Catholic and he came to find out that the Mexican immigrants were also Catholic. Slowly, within Kendal there developed a sense that he was "different" from the Mexicans and his grandparents for some "deep reason" that made it impossible for him to believe in God.

The therapist had also discovered in Kendal's Relational History that his father had beaten him with a belt and humiliated Kendal about his "weaknesses" for "not wanting to work hard." Kendal's identity as a young White "Rasta man" was fragile and insecure, and he protected it by belittling Devan's belief in God.

It was as though the internalized "weirdness" aspect of Kendal's early views of Mexicans and his French-speaking grandparents was unconsciously projected into Devan now. This fear of his own inferiority was at the root of his attacks on Devan's religion. And while Kendal feared that his attacks were "based in some kind of racism," they seemed motivated more by the ways he had felt isolated from his grandparents and humiliated or enraged by his father, than by skin color differences or other aspects of the Mexican farmers. Kendal's refusal to accept Devan's religion as "making sense" and needing his respect initiated Kendal's curiosity about his own racism. Unblocking revealed that his feelings of humiliation and isolation had fed into his desire to make fun of others who seemed "weird," and yet, he also identified as "being a weird Rasta." Devan felt compassionate and shocked to hear what Kendal said about his grandparents and his father in the Unblocking. They were then able to continue in Real Dialogue, to speak openly about their differences in religious beliefs and their fears of the effects of racism in the world around them.

★★★

The previous examples do not always include all the ways in which the other partner (the observer partner who was not interviewed) was already identifying with some of what had been projected, or was playing out defensively in the projected aspect. Time and space simply do not allow full descriptions of the back-and-forth dynamic of projective identification in couples in the WOC sessions of Dialogue Therapy. We hope the reader can imagine how the projected material of one partner is picked up and identified with by the other in such a way so as to keep the cycles of projective identifications rolling forward through years or decades of painful polarization and lack of intimacy or deadening vitality.

The Unblocking process is not reserved for one partner, even though some of the previous examples emphasize only one partner in the couple. Nor is this process used only once per partner. Sometimes Unblocking will be done several times in a single session. Dialogue Therapists use Unblocking whenever and as often as it seems warranted, spread over the course of the therapy as a whole.

Typically, the frequency of Unblocking declines as the partners become better at WOC and using Real Dialogue skills. In fact, partners take pride and eventually pleasure in being able to get through their own blocks together without therapist assistance. However, therapists may find they still use this technique, even in the follow-up session after the conclusion of the initial Dialogue Therapy process. Generally, Dialogue Therapists should try to keep the process of RD (through Coaching and Alter-Ego) going on between partners as much as possible and to convey to partners that it is their responsibility to open mindful spaces and get to know each other as individuals.

Clinicians who regularly conduct individual therapy may not see a difference between the Unblocking portion of Dialogue Therapy and typical psychodynamic psychotherapy. There are many overlaps, to be sure, but there are differences. Unblocking is used only in times when Real Dialogue breaks down. It is also used primarily to show partners how old experiences with important attachment figures can be "written on the body," indelibly imprinted on the limbic brain and, through projective identification, are repeated with their partner.

Refining a theory of relational blockages

To expand and refine a theory of relational blockages, we want to consider here some other couple therapies that focus on blocks, some research on blocks, along with another example of Dialogue Therapy's use of Unblocking. Janis Abrahms Spring (1996) writes about some common self-statements in partners which act as blocks to thinking and communication between them. She refers to them as "cognitive blocks" in that they seem to have their origins in another time and place that present problems in *current* thinking. The blocks only feel like blocks in the *couple relationship* (not when one is by oneself) and they are often attributed outside the self, as emanating from *the other*. This is one reason why partners' blocks in communication look like a control battle: "I want you to be different, and I won't be satisfied until you change into the form I envision or desire" or "I won't be satisfied until *I* have control over the way *you* are."[1]

The person who is unconscious or disowning of their own "shadow impulses" (to borrow some Jungian terminology) feels they have been wronged in some way and must go after the "criminal" – the *other person* – for a type of psychic justice. When an individual has a wish or impulse they cannot own, and they've *decided* (indeed, it feels like they *know*) that the other person is the one who has robbed them of their rightful stuff, stuff that allows that disowned impulse to be expressed, then they will engage in a battle royal with the putative transgressor, a battle as important as life versus death, because *psychically* it feels exactly that grave, that threatening, and that momentous to the individual.

Abrahms Spring (1996) has specialized in working with couples who have experienced infidelities, but many of her observations are apt for all couples having difficulty with projective identifications. Here are some examples of internal statements that set up relational blocks: "My partner should intuit what I need. I shouldn't have to spell it out" or "My partner hurt me, let me down, and they owe it to me to change first" or "I can't or shouldn't act in trust-enhancing ways when I'm so angry" or "If I have to ask for something, then it doesn't count." Many of these statements have their roots in early experiences with parents, sibs, or other important figures ("love objects" or attachment figures). Some of these notions are exemplified in the Unblocking vignettes.

In other words, certain states of mind – which usually feel like immovable facts or reality – belong to *other times and other realities* and to relationships with *other people*.

The latter can also be exemplified in the phenomenon of trans-generational transmission of anxieties and traumas, called "the telescoping of generations" (Faimberg, 2005). For example, family members from a generation growing up in a war zone may transfer inner worlds of anxiety, distrust, and revenge fantasies to the next generation, unconsciously and often wordlessly. A partner in a couple may feel certain anxieties, not identifying or understanding their true or original source, and then may attribute the reason for the anxiety to their partner, the person perhaps closest to them – confusing proximity with causality[2] – making the partner an "intimate enemy" (Young-Eisendrath, 2019). We see many examples of projective identification in this situation, an unconscious emotional "hijacking" of one partner by another, as described in Chapter 3.

Examples of projective identification in the couple Kathy and Bill emerged in our Unblocking interview with Kathy. Kathy and Bill were attempting a dialogue in the first WOC session in which Kathy was about to paraphrase something Bill had said, and she exclaimed: "I can't do this! It's too hard. I just want to explain myself, I can't say back what you're saying!" The co-therapists stopped the process and set up the Unblocking interview with Kathy, which has been condensed and excerpted below. In the following example, Kathy and Bill have found themselves at an impasse about, *prima facie*, the division of household chores. It becomes clearer, through the Unblocking with Kathy, that the chores, and in fact, any kind of commitment, accountability, or "pinning oneself down" to a time, place, task, etc., is tantamount to a complete loss of personal freedom in her mind. It is an experience of being thwarted, along with unavoidable unhappiness and pain, based on negative experiences she'd had with her parents.

JP: *So, Kathy, can you say a little about what was coming up for you there?*

K: *I was becoming frustrated that we were talking about making an "agreement" about family chores. I don't want anything to do with such a routinized way of doing things in the house.*

JP: *What happens for you when you imagine doing that?*

K: *I get really angry, and want to protest, or even leave!*

JP: *As in: "Leave Bill"?*

K: *Well, not really, but I want to escape the house, the rules, the drudgery . . .*

JP: *Because it means . . .?*

K: *That I'm not FREE! Or creative, or spontaneous, or playful, or able to just be myself.*

JP: *Do you have any thoughts about where you would get this idea?*
[Introducing the notion that, again, chores and lack of creativity, might not automatically or intrinsically be a cause of suffering – she *learned* this emotional connection.]

K: *Um . . . well . . . my father used to hate, absolutely hate, coming home and having to do chores after a long day at work. He really resented it whenever my mother who was a lovely, kind, and respectful person, would ask him to do anything on the domestic front. I mean, she worked too, but it was as if his work outside the home was more important than hers, and she was tying him down by asking anything of him regarding the household.*

JP: *And what was your relationship with your father like?*

[Trying to find a "transitive" connection: K identified with her father's experience.]

K: *I kind of adored him. I thought he was the best father. He had high standards – for work AND play. And he loved that he could make a life for us kids where we got to play a lot, do our own thing, especially outside. We spent a lotta time playing outside, I remember. He was proud of being able to provide that. That, and to be able to give us money when we got older. He took pride in that. He wanted us to be able to have the freedom to do what we wanted, and to afford it.*

The Unblocking interview proceeded with Kathy describing some of the feelings she would have, which were harder to bear, or even "know," because she could not reconcile them with her positive view of her father.

JP: *Your father would become irritable after a long day's work, giving you the sense he resented having to work for a living, being constrained somehow. He would rather have been free, and he didn't see himself as free in the context of home and housework . . . something in this mood and state of mind, which then would eventuate in him losing his temper, also scared you, alienated you, angered you. This admixture of feelings, both from the vantage point of your "child self," feeling threatened, and from the vantage point of your father (because you empathized with his irritation, resentment, and anger) is something you are trying to avoid in yourself at all costs. It takes too much energy. I wonder if it makes more sense to you to attribute the dysphoria, irritation, disappointment, and dissatisfaction to Bill – and that the creative, playful, spontaneous attributes stay with you? This might make you a bit fed up with Bill?*

JP continued to work with Kathy to identify what she would feel and think about Bill when she had to do "domestic things" in any kind of routine. It became clear that Bill was equivalent in her mind to her mother, setting boundaries and acting to inhibit her free expression, as her father used to attribute to her mother. At the same time, she may have been less conscious of expecting Bill to "provide for her" as her father did (she would have consciously found this notion quite distasteful), so that she could play more and be more spontaneous and unfettered. Kathy, in her identification with her father, was behaving as though Bill were a parental figure keeping her child-self from completely free expression; she protested when he would make requests or try to negotiate an agreement with her as an equal – *as if* he were unilaterally, in an authoritarian manner, laying down the law or making a demand on her. Bill would become her intimate enemy at such moments. Bill, as part of a projective identification, began to feel that Kathy was immature, and that he was the only one in the family who could be expected to sustain "adult" concerns and functions. He began to feel especially irritable, "un-free" and uncreative himself – he who had grown up with extremely free-spirited parents, an irony (which is likely no more than a set of projective identifications) that was lost on both of these partners until they worked in the Unblocking process. They reported that they would become blocked in their decision making, especially about becoming parents. And because they tended to avoid arguing, they had become shut down in their relationship.

★★★

The loss of liveliness (or the deadness of intimacy and curiosity) is just one difficulty couples report when they come to couple therapy, and it manifests especially in blocked communication (Johnson, 2008; Gottman & Schwartz-Gottman, 2015; Perel, 2006, 2017). Johnson (2008) describes some of the most frequent "Demon Dialogues," as she calls them, for example:

She labels them "Find the Bad Guy," "the Protest Polka," and "Freeze and Flee." In Find the Bad Guy the partners are fighting for self-protection when there is a feeling of vulnerability or hurt, and each one blames the other for the pain they are experiencing. Each individual becomes so preoccupied with *self*-protection that they cannot hear the *other* partner's pain or distress and its corresponding logic. In the Protest Polka one partner is looking for any kind of response from the other partner. And when there is none forthcoming "We . . . protest," states Johnson, because "attachment relationships are the only ties on Earth where *any* response is better than none" (p. 74). The "Protest Polka" is subtler, harder to recognize; it creates a more stable loop than "Find the Bad Guy" where attacks reign and are easier to peg. In the "Protest Polka," one partner seems demanding, or as though they are actively protesting the experience of disconnection, while the other protests the implied criticism being leveled at them by withdrawing and quietly or passively going against the first partner in some way. One partner reaches out, usually through criticism, and the other retreats, feeling stung. And the pursuer-distancer pattern repeats itself, creating a negative experience for the couple, a "stable indefiniteness." Gottman's (1994) research shows that many couples stuck in this pattern of non-responsiveness separate before their fifth anniversary.

In Johnson's third Demon Dialogue "Freeze and Flee", the therapist may sense a "dead tension" or "tense deadness" where neither partner seems invested in the relationship and they appear to be frozen and shut down, trying to exhibit no feeling or need. Couples in this state may look polite and cooperative, but there is really a sense of them having "given up" on hoping, or fighting, for the relationship. Bill and Kathy exhibited a mild version of this latter pattern in their chronic illnesses, depression, and avoidance of certain conflicts.

These are also examples of some patterns that will emerge and re-emerge as couples work on their dialogue skills. The patterns are usually recapitulations of the couple's initial complaints, or the reasons they reported for coming to Dialogue Therapy in the first place.

The identification of parent–child complexes in partners is relatively straightforward most of the time in Dialogue Therapy, but it is noteworthy when there is "love between equals" that another type of complex can be easily activated – namely that of siblings (Young-Eisendrath, 2019). The importance of sibling relationships in determining aspects of couple relating is too often overlooked in clinical literature. Sibling relationships, or fantasied sibling relationships (the putative sibling or no-sibling in only children, adopted children, twins, a few examples to consider) also play a role in the ways partners enter into projective identification.

Many issues related to competition, sharing of attention and other emotional, or narcissistic resources, envy, responsibility, and protectiveness arise in couples as part of a sibling transference that can also be observed at times in the individual therapy context between a therapist and a client. In Dialogue Therapy, e.g. a client reported that when it came to her partner's view of her she was "always Cinder-fucking-ella," left at home from the ball. He was always one of the "lucky" stepsisters. While these dynamics could also have Oedipal derivatives, they were much more easily understood through the partner's sibling relationships, explored in Unblocking. As all Dialogue Therapists come to see, Unblocking is one of the best tools in our tool kit. It is used to get the couple back on the track of Real Dialogue so that they can gain the skills they need, but it also provides the rich opportunity for partners to gain specific and lasting insights into their own (and each other's) emotional landscapes, as differentiated adults.

Notes

1 See, for instance: Gariepy-Boutin and Maas' (2017) review of Paul Denis' concept of "emprise": a type of control of the other.
2 See Freud's (1915a, 1915b) description of associative reasoning.

Bibliography

Barrett, L.F. (2017). *How Emotions Are Made: The Secret Life of the Brain*. New York: Houghton-Mifflin Harcourt.

DeKoven, F.M., Goldman, R.N. & Siegel, J.P. (2020, June 16). "Couple impasses: Three therapeutic approaches." *Clinical Social Work Journal*, 1–14, https://doi.org/10.1007/s10615-020-00764-x.

Denis, P. (2017). "Emprise et satisfaction." *Presentation at Vermont Association for Psychoanalytic Studies Annual Meeting*, Burlington, VT.

Faimberg, H. (2005). *The Telescoping of Generations: Listening to the Narcissistic Link between Generations*. London: Routledge.

Fonagy, P., Gyorgy, G., Jurist, E. & Target, M. (2004). *Affect Regulation, Mentalization, and the Development of the Self*. New York: Other Press.

Freud, S. (1915a). "Instincts and their Vicissitudes." *The Standard Edition of the Complete Psychological Works of Sigmund Freud*, Vol. 14, James Strachey (Ed.), 117–140. London: Hogarth Press.

————. (1915b). "The Unconscious." *The Standard Edition of the Complete Psychological Works of Sigmund Freud*, Vol. 14, James Strachey (Ed.), 159–215. London: Hogarth Press.

Gottman, J. (1994). *Why Marriages Succeed or Fail . . . And How You Can Make Yours Last*. New York: Simon & Schuster.

Gottman, J. & Schwartz-Gottman, J. (2015). *10 Principles for Doing Effective Couples Therapy*. New York: W.W. Norton & Company.

Johnson, S. (2008). *Hold Me Tight: Seven Conversations for a Lifetime of Love*. New York: Little, Brown and Company.

Lachmann, F.M. & Lichtenberg, J. (1992). "Model scenes: Implications for psychoanalytic treatment." *Journal of the American Psychoanalytic Association*, 40, 117–137.

Lichtenberg, J., Lachmann, F. & Fosshage, J.L. (2016). *Self and Motivational Systems: Toward A Theory of Psychoanalytic Technique*. New York: Routledge.

Mitchell, J. (2003). *Siblings: Sex and Violence*. Malden, MA: Blackwell Publishing.

Perel, E. (2006). *Mating in Captivity: Unlocking Erotic Intelligence*. New York: HarperCollins.

Perel, E. (2017). *The State of Affairs: Rethinking Infidelity*. New York: Harper.

Slavin, M.O. & Kriegman, D. (1992). *The Adaptive Design of the Human Psyche: Psychoanalysis, Evolutionary Biology, and the Therapeutic Process*. New York: Guilford.

Spring, J.A. (1996). *After the Affair: Healing the Pain and Rebuilding Trust When a Partner Has Been Unfaithful*. New York: Harper Collins.

Young-Eisendrath, P. (2019). *Love Between Equals: Relationship as a Spiritual Path*. Boulder, CO: Shambala.

9 Role Reversal, Wrap-Ups, and Six-month Follow-up

One of the pillars supporting Dialogue Therapy is empathy, as described in Chapter 4. Empathy is an attitude, and a skill, involving the grasp of another person's experience, their pain and emotional meanings, and "feeling into" them while also being able to hold onto one's own subjectivity, one's own mind. Empathy, in fact, requires a mindful gap or space between one's own emotional and cognitive experience and the other's. This means that we must see, hear, and feel the other person in such a way that the other person can validate that we have "got it." We are not simply projecting or identifying with the other when we are truly empathic.

In projection, we "cover" the other person with our own experiences, which may be unconscious or semi-conscious. In *identification*, we take on the other's experiences as our own or we become like them, even though that likeness may be unconscious (for example, you might not enjoy your father's critical nature, but you might become just like him in being critical). By contrast, empathy includes an ongoing experience of separate subjectivities while being able to see things through the other person's eyes, from the other's vantage points, and even being able to apprehend the other person's logic and conclusions, given their experience and assumptions. Empathy is also not the same as *agreement* (even though agreement *may* be one discovery of an empathic connection). Empathy is simply knowing, and perhaps expressing, what it is *like to be the other person* while holding onto and respecting one's own individuality or signature of meanings.

Role Reversal

As couples progress through the steps of Dialogue Therapy and begin to use Real Dialogue skillfully for Working on a Conflict at home, as well as in sessions, the Dialogue Therapists introduce them to a capstone exercise, coming from psychodrama. This exercise increases understanding and builds empathy for oneself and one's partner: Role Reversal (RR). This intervention is usually introduced around the third or fourth session of DT in the co-therapist model, and in the twelfth to fourteenth hour in the solo model. The Role Reversal takes (both partners) a minimum of two hours, whether in the solo or co-therapist approach – thirty minutes of RR with a partner, then some

DOI: 10.4324/9781003200840-9

exploration of the effects on the listening partner, including observations of what was seen and heard.

The process is then repeated with the other partner, followed again by Real Dialogue about what happened. There is a Wrap-Up at the end of the two-hour RR session in the co-therapist model, and a Wrap-Up at the end of each one-hour RR session in the solo model.

The Role Reversal consists of the following: therapists begin by telling the couple that "we will be doing something a bit different today. We'll start with some dialogue, and move to another task, which will be described at the time we shift." After the opening of the session – listening to the couple decide on a topic for WOC – the therapist(s) should listen for a point of emotional contact or conflict that would be ripe or rich for empathic investigation. As Dialogue Therapists gain experience and mastery of the DT process, they will develop a good ear for hearing the kind of issue that is likely to blossom in RR. But almost any issue will produce some good insights and outcomes. The point at which the therapist hears such an issue, the therapist says: "We are going to do another activity (or exercise) now, which I will describe in a moment. Right now I am going to change chairs with X (the partner who is going into the RR)." The set up requires the therapist to switch chairs with one partner.

In the co-therapist model, the interviewee will be that therapist's typical interviewee. In the solo model, the therapist will interview the partner who seems more affectively moved or charged by the topic (see Figure 9.1). Then the therapist says: "This interview is called Role Reversal, and it gives us an opportunity to observe your empathy for your partner, to see how accurately you perceive your partner. I am going to interview you as though you *were* your partner, calling you by your partner's name. You do not have to act or sound like your partner, although you can do that if you would like. For now, I would like you to step into your partner's shoes and answer my questions as you think your partner would. I will address you by your partner's name. Do not look at your partner for any clues. If you do not know something, don't revert to your own identity, but just say 'I don't know.' You are not expected to know all the answers to the questions, but guessing is very

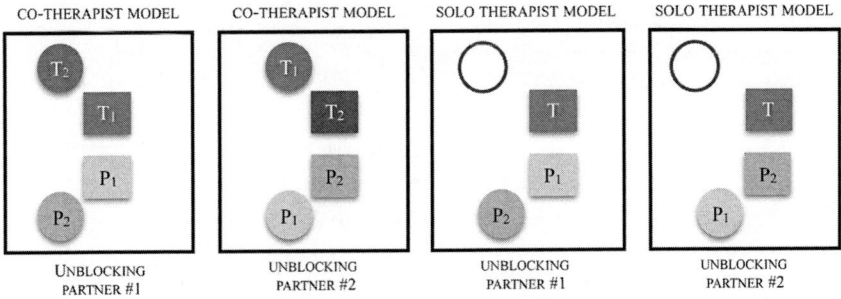

Figure 9.1 Solo model

welcome. Do you understand the instructions?" If instructions need to be repeated or fleshed out, then that happens until the interviewee is entirely on board with the setup.

The therapist then begins, often picking up a thread from what the couple was just discussing. The therapist can ask questions that arise from their own curiosity, or elaborate on what the partners were just speaking about. As the interviewer proceeds, they should use Real Dialogue to reflect and remain interested in the subjective experience. For example, if the partner says "Well, I still don't feel confident about my attractiveness as a woman because sometimes I am afraid that I'm not in good shape or athletic enough," then the therapist may say something like, "So, you're saying that you don't like the way you look and feel in your own body, as a woman – is that it?" And if that is confirmed, then the therapist may say: "Tell me more about that. How does that interfere with your sexual intimacy, for example?" An experienced Dialogue Therapist can become very playful in this exercise and can reach back over the earlier sessions and bring up something by surprise about the other partner. For instance, the therapist might say: "XX (partner's name), I recall you saying in the second session of Working on a Conflict that you really don't like to spend money. Can you tell me more about that and why you prefer being frugal?" This is a surprise to the interviewee because it wasn't connected in an immediate way to the topic that brought about the initiation of the RR.

Many intricate topics can enter into a Role Reversal. For example, with Bill and Kathy, the therapists were able to explore aspects of the failed decision-making about becoming parents in a way that was unexplored and even avoided in the WOC sessions. And so, RR can very much deepen the ability of each partner to see, hear, and feel into the experience of the other.

And yet, there are some standard questions that should be included in each RR session, to be asked at any point during the half-hour RR interview, which are in the therapists' "tool bag" and are to be brought out if there is a lull or sense of running out of steam. It is important to ask the standard questions at some point in the interview, but they can be asked in any order and blended into any topic. These questions are as follows:

1   If you had a magic wand and could change one thing about yourself, XX (partner's name), what would it be?
2   If you could change one thing about your partner, XX, what would it be?
3   What do you like best/most about yourself, XX?
4   What do you like best/most about your partner, XX?
5   How do you feel about your sex life with your partner, XX?
6   How do you feel about your partner as a parent (if there is a child or children), XX?
7   Where do you want to be five years from now in this relationship, XX?

After each RR interview, the listening partner returns to their seat across from their partner. The partners are then back to "being themselves."

The therapist then asks the listening partner to offer feedback and reflections on what they experienced. Partners are asked to use Real Dialogue to speak and respond, as well as to remain curious and ask questions about why the partner said or thought certain things about the listener. Some important aspects of this reflection include letting their partner know how accurately they felt they were portrayed, how they seemed to be represented in their partner's mind (through the role play), and what it was like for them to be depicted by their partner. Typically the listening partner feels gratitude, and even pleasure, in hearing the Role Reversal.

In the co-therapy model, often there is also time for Reflecting Team interactions with the co-therapist. In the co-therapy approach, the other therapist and partner "pair," then become the new RR pair and the process is repeated. A Wrap-Up is offered at the end of this two-hour session.

In the solo model, typically the RR happens in two sessions: first with partner #1 and then with partner #2. At the end of each session, the therapist shares their observations and insights about what they saw in the whole RR process. This is done in the Wrap-Up at the end of the hour.

The Role Reversal is an opportunity for insights into non-rational levels of expression and often non-verbal experiences between the partners. Role Reversal also allows therapists to know more about how closely each partner has observed and understood the other. Do they seem to accurately understand each other in more or less equal measure, or is there a large discrepancy between them in who truly observes and understands?

This is important information for the couple and the therapists to learn. Early in our careers, in our experiences as family and couple therapists, another exercise called Trading Places was often used (see, e.g., Young-Eisendrath, 1984). When this exercise occurred in couple therapy, the couple traded places with the therapists, "becoming" couple therapists while the therapists played the couple being treated. In family therapy, trading places often involved children trading places with parents and each playing the role of the other. Trading Places often brought lightness, laughter, and fascination to the therapy environment – which then served to decrease defensiveness and playfully introduce empathic resonance for all parties. Like Trading Places, Role Reversal can echo the ways in which projections and projective identifications were first *developed* or *acquired* in a couple; this echo, or parallel process, makes WOC and Real Dialogue more effective. Typically, partners find that Role Reversal is both challenging (making them "sweat") and creative (being fun) in ways that deepen what they have learned in WOC sessions.

The session Wrap-Up for RR in both the co-therapy and solo approaches includes the therapists' observations of the role play, noting how easy or difficult it seemed for partners to play each other, or any insights they seem to (or reported to) have achieved through RR.

The Wrap-Up

Every Dialogue Therapy session concludes with a Wrap-Up, which takes about 10–15 minutes in the co-therapy model and 5–10 minutes in the solo model. After completing the task(s) of the session (e.g., Evaluation, Working on a Conflict, Role Reversal), the therapist or therapists form a circle with the partners or pull their chairs together so that everyone can see everyone else face-to-face (see Figure 9.2). The Wrap-Up helps partners transition to the time and space outside the therapy set-up, and to remember and internalize what they should be taking home to practice and to understand more fully. Wrap-Up gives each partner a sense of what the therapists have observed and understood (or hypothesized) about the "snags" in partners' relating to each other, and the projective identifications causing those snags. Through the Wrap-Up, again therapists use Real Dialogue: speaking for themselves, checking out whether they are understood, and finding out if the partners "got" what the therapists have said.

In the Wrap-Up, the therapists (in both the solo and co-therapy model) talk about what they have learned about the couple in that session, offer some psycho-education or other literature or research that is applicable to the particular session. Sometimes, *Love Between Equals* (Young-Eisendrath, 2019), *Real Dialogue: The Skill* videos (Vols. 1, 2, 3), TED Talks, and assessments of adult attachment styles may be "assigned." Most of these are not exactly "homework," but more like suggestions that may or may not be incorporated. The only true *homework* for Dialogue Therapy is learning Real Dialogue and reading the mini booklets (Appendix B) that are used to teach it. On occasion, if the therapists feel the clients can skillfully apply them, the terms "projection" and "projective identification" are introduced and defined.

Within these explanations, the therapists also describe *where* and *how* they recognize these phenomena operating between the partners. They give specific

Wrap-Up

CO-THERAPIST MODEL   SOLO THERAPIST MODEL

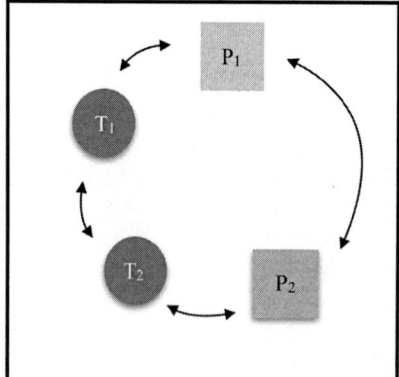
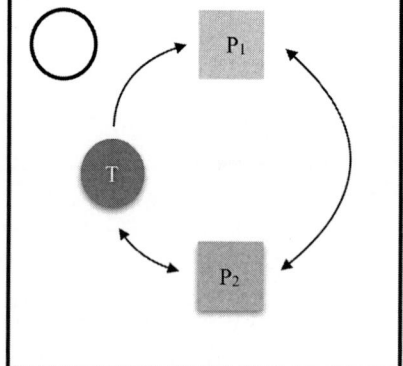

Figure 9.2 Therapist and partners face-to-face

examples for the couple to consider, based on the material shared in the present session. The formal terms are not necessary for the therapists to describe and problematize the painful, repetitive patterns in the couple's relating, and why those patterns might recycle, i.e., what seems to stimulate certain emotional habits and reactions in each partner toward the other, alongside the confusion and sense of alienation.

In the Wrap-Up after the Evaluation Session(s), the therapist(s) also include the reasons why the partners seem to be a good fit for Dialogue Therapy, where the conflict(s) between them seem to present obstacles, and why that appears to be happening as part of a projective process.

Therapists may also introduce the idea that partners come from different "tribes" or family cultures. Barack Obama once described, in a public talk, his nuclear family dynamics in terms of "the round-faced, fierce, meat-eating and hunting tribe" (to characterize Michelle and daughter Sasha), while calling himself and daughter Melia, the "long-faced, peaceful, vegetarian, gatherer tribe." He was using humor to talk about differences in his family. Sometimes partners' different cultures have their own sets of rules, values, prescriptions and proscriptions that are hidden and unconscious, creating the "different packages that love came in." These different packages may stir positive feelings for one partner, and puzzle or stun the other.

In the Wrap-Up, therapists summarize differences and give an overview of how or why they may be contributing to the projections and projective identifications.

Here's a clinical example of a Wrap-Up in a couple described in Chapter 8:

THERAPIST: Charlie, you have believed that someone going off to relax was merely a cover for that person becoming compromised or incapacitated in their functioning, via alcohol abuse. You would then feel abandoned and betrayed and not cared for. You expressed your anger about this through sarcasm and other indirect means that allowed you to let off steam, even as you knew it wouldn't get you very far. Your own direct requests never got you what you needed. Now, whenever Barbara needs time to herself to recharge, it is as if she is *lying* to you about some awful secret and is *abandoning* you – not simply taking care of herself with a rest. Barbara, you have *absorbed Charlie's fears* and old betrayals as a personal failure on your part, and have *capitulated to his unconscious demands* in these moments, not allowing for your own enjoyment. Once the two of you became curious about the experiences from other times, places and relationships, and began asking directly about each other's subjective experiences, you realized expressing needs could be much more direct, simple, and not personalized.

Another example Wrap-Up is from the case of Ellen and Josh:

THERAPIST: Ellen, you had at least one powerful experience of trying to comfort a loved one who was very important to you, a man who was vulnerable and in pain – and being rejected. You felt as though your comforts were inadequate to his pain. That humiliation has been displaced in time, carried to your relationship with Josh, and has you *anticipating his rejection whenever he is in need of comfort*; you have developed ways to preemptively reject *him* before he can hurt you. And he has indeed felt hurt, and has pulled away from you, leaving you to feel even more abandoned and disconnected from him – working against what you are conscious of deeply desiring, but also giving you a sense of control. Josh, you have *identified with this rejection* and have felt either *more* vulnerable, or avoidant of interaction with Ellen, working against what *you* desire, but also giving you the illusion of control. You have both learned through the Unblocking and Real Dialogue, that things are not as they "seem," once you inquire into each other's subjective experience, and understand the other's vantage point. You cannot assume you know what the other person is making of your expressions until you ask, and until you learn how the other person has come to associate certain expressions with pain or trauma. You have learned, through RD, that it pays to ask, to listen closely, and be able to accurately reflect back to your partner what they are trying to express. Each partner's appreciation for this is immeasurable.

The Wrap-Up in the final DT session

The final (technically penultimate, but final in the first process) Dialogue Therapy session, in the co-therapist approach, typically occurs in the sixth two-hour meeting, and in the solo model, it typically occurs in the fourteenth, fifteenth, or sixteenth hour. By the time of the final DT session, the partners should be at least somewhat skillful in using the Real Dialogue techniques, and have used them at home to work through conflicts. We often find that, by this time, which is roughly six to seven months into the treatment in the co-therapist model, and around eight months for the solo model, partners can use RD skillfully in the presence of the therapist within a session and report using outside, as well. Dialogue Therapists look for three aspects of "working through" projective identifications through RD: (1) willingness of partners to use RD skills in session, without being reminded either by the therapist or by the partner; (2) the ability to move through conflict and negotiation with a degree of autonomy in which each partner seems to "get" the skills; (3) an ability to talk about difficult topics (such as loss or fears) without reverting back to active or passive aggression and splitting.

In the "final" session before the six months break, we have noted some different patterns in couples: some partners "pick fights" and seem to regress to earlier sessions; some appear quieter than usual; some (even many) are pleased and satisfied they have developed skills and abilities they have not had before.

The prospect of not having regular contact with a Dialogue Therapist (with scheduled sessions on the calendar) any longer – and perhaps now having new "date nights" instead of therapy (see Nick Hornby's book and BBC series, *State of the Union*, for a light treatment of this kind of thing), partners and couples may feel either afraid or confident about being on their own without the container of DT.

The Dialogue Therapists continue in this session to help the couple talk about ways to adjust, refine, and adapt the Real Dialogue format they have been using in the consulting room, all with the intention of facilitating partners' creation of a context for changing the ways they Witness and communicate with each other – *in the absence of the therapists*. In this session, Dialogue Therapists may touch on typical pitfalls couples experience or on the particular obstacles faced.

Dialogue Therapists also discuss the ways in which partners might prepare for or anticipate roadblocks, as well as some pathways out of these difficult situations. In the final Wrap-Up, Dialogue Therapists may engage in any or all of the following:

1 Reminding partners of the resource of individual psychotherapy for working with emotional themes discovered in DT that remain raw or distressing.
2 Recognizing the signs of projective identifications that can lead to making an "intimate enemy" of your partner and using RD and emotional warmth when those signs come up.
3 Reinstating a mindful gap to return to curiosity.
4 Holding in mind one's own dignity and remembering that shame and humiliation breed impulses to run and hide or to become enraged, neither of which bring about desired intimacy or understanding.
5 Knowing that, on occasion, taking a short break from overheated conversation, with a promise for later connection (a "time certain"), can actually *preserve* RD skills and the possibility of negotiation.
6 Accepting that it is not the job of partners to *make each other happy*.

These suggestions are general and any couple can use one or all of them. However, in the last session (before the six-month break) Wrap-Up, Dialogue Therapists also always offer a personalized summary for the particular couple – with that couple's unique idioms, projective identifications, and other themes of what has been learned over the course of the meetings.

In the following example, with our demonstration couple, Bill and Kathy, the therapists offered these comments as one portion of the final Wrap-Up (which included several other observations and issues):

PYE: *Dialogue Therapy has helped you see yourselves as individuals, and as different from each other, and to not be afraid of those differences, but instead, to be interested in them. So here are some differences we've seen between the two of you. Kathy, you come from a family that can help you out financially, as an adult, and it sort of frames your life so that you're not afraid about money. But you also saw your father irritated and annoyed about having to work so hard for the family's money, and be the breadwinner, so there are some leftovers from that, which have to do with your desire to protect your freedom. You have come to the conclusion that freedom depends (as in, you can ask your father for it) on money and you just expect you will always have plenty of money. This is not a universe in which Bill shares. Bill, in your tribe, it was more like: not having money was what gave people freedom. So . . . in your relationship money does not carry a single meaning that you two share − it is not a single meaning to both of you. So when you talk about it, you are not talking about the same thing, and you must ask and listen to each other about those different meanings. It won't help you to then judge each other that one of you is not doing it the right, or true, way.*

JP: *Kathy, if your dad was so frustrated by having to work so much, and seemed kind of "mad at the world" for having to do that, then you might've made an equivalency in your mind between working and unhappiness, and you would not want any of that. One thing you might do, then, is "give away" to Bill the idea that work equals unhappiness, and then Bill actually takes that identity on, looking and acting quite unhappy with his situation, not very much fun, but also as though he is not a very strong person who provides for others. It puts you in a position of holding the freedom-equals-fun equation, and feeling resentful of Bill.*

PYE: *And Bill, your family, it seems, idealized a certain kind of freedom from the physical world, valuing only the metaphysical, as you have said. But the life your family led, outside more traditional community, may not have given you some of the skills you would've liked to learn, to cope with the larger world. So, it is a conflicted experience for you to be working in a more traditional job or schedule, providing for you and Kathy, while you idealize and envy her freedom and her metaphysical approach to life. You cannot imagine that you also have that in you, i.e., you have "given that away" to her. But then, you resent her for it when it comes to things like household chores that just need to be done. So, we have seen the two of you get stuck in your relating when these different ways of understanding money feel threatening to the two of you.*

JP: *Through the Working on a Conflict sessions, you have been able to see that you can keep talking through these experiences of difference, and not feel as threatened as you had been in the past. Through practicing Real Dialogue, you have learned to not take your differences as personal referenda, or a competition, and you have allowed yourselves to become more curious and empathic about the differences and their origins. You have learned more about these origins and their logic from the Unblocking exercises, and have developed greater empathy for each other through the Role Reversals. Your idealizations of all things metaphysical has diminished, allowing the two of you to become more friendly and cooperative with each other about sharing household work, family planning decisions, and the pursuit of your own creative impulses.*

The therapists then make plans to follow up with the couple for a session in six months. Another part of the final session before the six-month "break" includes giving a rationale for such a break, and the reasons for meeting again at the six-month mark.

The knowledge that they will be coming back to the therapists at a later date can help couples feel the liberty of testing and using their internalizations of the Real Dialogue skills, while also knowing that there will be a definite future contact with the therapists. That knowledge, we propose, helps couples to continue feeling the background containment of the structure of Dialogue Therapy, while becoming independent of the therapy sessions. There is also a kind of "deadline" when they will show up to an actual DT session to have their skills assessed. Most couples anticipate the six-month follow-up in a positive way. Dialogue Therapists also say, "We are still in the process of Dialogue Therapy. You just are not seeing the therapist(s) during this time, but you can certainly call and make an appointment if you need an extra session or two during this hiatus." This hiatus also implies the therapists' faith in the couples' abilities to use the skills and insights they have gained.

The six-month follow-up session

The follow-up session occurs approximately six months after Dialogue Therapy ends. This session begins in the manner of previous Working on a Conflict sessions, with the couple being asked to talk to each other about "what they want to focus on in this session." There are several purposes for this session: (1) to study the way the couple has been able to implement (or not) the Real Dialogue skills and insights from DT into their lives; (2) to help the couple make any refinements or adjustments in their use of the RD and DT; (3) to boost the couple's confidence and competence in using skills and insights gained, and to steer the couple back to the domain of the RD skills; and (4) to hear feedback and evaluate the outcomes of the therapy for the longer term. If the couple needs more help from actual sessions of DT (because of any number of issues), then the Dialogue Therapist will suggest one or two more meetings during the Wrap-Up. Readings, videos, TED talks, or other resources may also be suggested if they can support the couple further in integrating their skills and insights.

If the couple has made good use of the Dialogue Therapy in the interim, and they have internalized its lessons, then one or both of the partners might say that they are only meeting because they "have to," as part of the DT model, but do not feel there is anything happening between them that they cannot manage themselves.

If the therapists have any doubts about the couple's abilities, then, to paraphrase Young-Eisendrath (1984), they "poke around like the family doctor" to see if a problem is lurking, hidden, or masked, that can be fairly easily activated. The therapists can then observe how well that re-activation is managed by the partners through RD. If the DT has worked well, the six-month follow-up session should have an anti-climactic feel, or even be a little dull, a quiet postscript. The topic in the follow-up is chosen by the couple, as in all WOC sessions unless there has been an infidelity or painful betrayal and then those issues must be addressed, as they would be if discovered in the Evaluation.

Typically, the follow-up session goes well and partners seem satisfied with the changes they have made, as well as confident about retaining them. If that is not the case, then, as we previously said, the Dialogue Therapist suggests one or two more sessions to "boost" the effects of the treatment.

The Wrap-Up at the time of follow-up, just as the Wrap-Up at the end of the six months, is also an opportunity for Dialogue Therapists to use Real Dialogue skills to explore and understand what partners may say critically or negatively about their experiences within the process of the therapy.

Therapists being honest with themselves, and with the clients, about their assessments of relative success or failure, affords all the individuals involved a certain dignity, respect, and appreciation. It also demonstrates the values espoused in the Dialogue Therapy and Real Dialogue endeavor.

Our aim in this follow-up session, especially in its Wrap-Up, is to end the work with the couple in ways that reinforce their sense of *working together* as differentiated individuals now, and also as having a promising "future" together in coming to see, hear, and feel each other freshly again and again – with renewed curiosity and mystery about what might evolve between them, whether in health or sickness, in wealth or poverty. Replacing the traditional wedding vows in today's "marriage between equals" is the recognition of the couple as a unique emotional space in which each person's growth and development can be welcomed and respected as the years and decades unfold. This is the promise of today's marriage, as well as the promise of Dialogue Therapy.

Bibliography

Young-Eisendrath, P. (1984). *Hags and Heroes: A Feminist Approach to Jungian Psychotherapy with Couples*. Toronto: Inner City Books.

Young-Eisendrath, P. (2019). *Love Between Equals: Relationship as a Spiritual Path*. Boulder, CO: Shambala.

10 Real Dialogue for opposing sides

Skill, method, and practice of facilitating difficult conversations outside of psychotherapy

When Dialogue Therapy was invented it was clear to the originators that projective identification was the obstacle to be overcome in repetitive, dangerous conflicts. At that time, we thought especially about bringing DT outside of the consulting room as a method to alleviate conflicts involving racism, sexism, and other equity issues. A great deal has changed from those early days of feminism and anti-racism when DT was coming on stage in the mid-1980s. Now, there are multiple dangerous polarizations and fragmentations in our societies, and in the world at large, that call for new ways of dealing with tense differences between us. There is no doubt that polarizations are the byproducts of chronic projections and projective identifications that express and evoke unconscious implications, meanings, and splits between people and groups.

Nonviolent communication and conflict resolution have not been able to settle down our most disruptive interactive hostilities. If they had, then we would be behaving better in our estrangements and disputes. For example, there are now brutal disputes about free speech, anti-racism, climate change, the safety of vaccines, health and sovereignty over one's body, sexual transgressions, and an ever-increasing variety of identity issues. Most of these are handled publicly through criticizing or blaming another or others. In our contemporary "calling out" culture, the conversation usually begins with blame and attack, so there's little to no chance for emotional containment and Witnessing. At best, one side is defensive and self-protective; at worst, both sides leave the conversation or act out with physical or psychological aggression directed against each other. Moral superiority, which can itself be a result of trauma, may be embraced in victimhood and can lead the victim to feel justified in attacking another person. This kind of engagement cannot lead to dialogue or repair. It can only lead to fractured relationships and increased alienation and attacks.

It now seems as though families, organizations, societies, and cultures are filled with polarizations, with moral superiority on all sides, further "empowered" by feelings of *disgust* that can readily lead to dehumanizing one's opponents. Most of us would say that we want more than anything to avoid a civil or international war, but unless we learn the ways to step outside chronic projective identification and the humiliation-rage cycle, and to recognize that our "enemies" are also human, we may be drawn into such wars. Before we

DOI: 10.4324/9781003200840-10

look at Real Dialogue as a method for dealing with difficult conversations, let's take a step back and look at our context.

First, the term "difficult conversations" typically means those conversations in which people disrespect and insult each other, and so they rarely get around to any kind of actual conversation about whatever the two sides are. Everything turns into accusation, insult, dispute, or defense. Often, each party feels humiliated and enraged. As we have seen, the experience of humiliation, the *perceived lowering of one's social status*, triggers a rage reaction (although the rage may not be expressed). Human beings naturally protect their social status in groups (and a couple can be considered a "group" in this context). This means they will defend and protect themselves at times when they feel their status is threatened, or, possibly with feelings of disgust, they will quit the interaction. In such situations, they will promote only their own arguments and evidence.

As humans, we do not have much subjective freedom when we *feel humiliated* because it is in *our nature* to protect and promote our survival and welfare, especially in a group. When we feel shamed by another, we are loath to roll over and show the soft underbelly of our vulnerability. When we are locked into chronic projective identifications in times of the humiliation-rage cycle, or influenced by disgust and moral superiority, we engage in repetitions of the same cycle of accusations and counter-accusations with emotional overtones that imply the other person is an enemy or is "toxic" (meaning non-human).

Unique characteristics of Real Dialogue

Throughout the decades of Dialogue Therapy's development, it has become ever clearer that projection of one's "enemy" into the other person is the first step on the path to objectifying that person. Further, conscious or unconscious feelings of being *morally superior* as a "victim" may color our perceptions with *disgust* and lead us to perceive that other person as "toxic" – a *thing* to be avoided or vanquished. When projective identifications are infused with disgust and moral superiority, they dehumanize others and become deeply disturbing. Think here about the "calling out" culture, for example, and disputes in the #MeToo movement, or other kinds of arguments about people feeling dismissed or harmed. Within these kinds of conversations or interactions it is impossible even to use the *rules* of conflict resolution, when no resolution or reconciliation is desired. In Real Dialogue, however, we make it abundantly clear to the parties involved that we are not aiming our facilitation toward the goals of reconciliation, balance, or resolution of the conflict. Instead, our objective is *respectful conflict and the ability to see, hear, and feel* both self and other within the conflict.

In the past couple of years, we have been teaching Real Dialogue as a *method* of co-facilitated conversation to non-mental health professionals (such as life coaches, leaders, mediators, executive coaches, and the like) so that they may facilitate difficult conversations outside of therapy settings. In such settings, the two warring parties must learn to see, hear, and feel each other accurately, and thus *humanize* each other, so that they can lower the levels of emotional threat and take in each other's words. Then, the two parties can begin to discover whether they have any common ground. Having and retaining deep and abiding differences between oneself and another, or others, is *wholly acceptable* as long as the differences are not used primarily to blame, shame, or dismiss the others.

Because of our snow globes of subjectivity, we see, hear, and feel things individually, each from our own world. Of course, most human societies (90–95%) have been at war since *Homo sapiens* have been on earth. We have little legacy of trusting anyone outside our own tribe. Conflicts between tribes have seemed relentlessly destructive, and war can seem inevitable. And yet, Real Dialogue has led us to believe that resolving, dissolving, or reducing the impact of projective identification has the potential for eliminating war – replacing it with facilitated and structured dialogue until the two parties experience themselves as fully human (subjective beings), no matter their differences, without trying to approach any agreement or solution. As cognitive science helps us to understand and accept that we do not inhabit "the same world," we may gain a greater respect for our differences and become more appreciative of drawing on all sides of a question or issue, so that we can use our natural human capacities for debate and argument to their best ends. As humans, we need to see, hear, and feel opposing sides on every issue because our individual experiences are so narrow and inadequate.

Real Dialogue is a skill (with three components) and a method. You already know the three components (*Speaking for Yourself*, *Listening Mindfully*, and *Remaining Curious*). They are used as methods for facilitating difficult conversations. They reduce the harmful and destructive dynamics of projective identifications and their implied threats. As in Dialogue Therapy, RD's desired outcome is greater differentiation and respect between parties, not greater agreement or reconciliation.

In other words, Real Dialogue is about humanizing conversational partners and allowing the two people to see, hear, and feel each other accurately, becoming witnesses through their debate. As cognitive scientist Donald Hoffman (2019) points out, because human reason is a method of *social persuasion* and not a search for truth, we humans must dispute and debate our empirical, scientific, value-laden opinions and perspectives. That is the only way we arrive at something close to the truth.

Real Dialogue: skill and method

The *skill* of Real Dialogue is the core aspect of the *method*, but it may or may not be learned by those clients who enter into a co-facilitated conversation, as participants, with Real Dialogue Specialists. If the facilitation happens only once or twice, then the participants may not learn the skill (during the actual intervention) despite being Coached, Facilitated, Doubled, and Unblocked in the processes of Speaking for Yourself, Listening Mindfully, and Remaining Curious, during the intervention.

To say this another way: the skill of Real Dialogue is *a self-improvement skill*, developed by learning and practicing the three components that we have been describing as RD in Dialogue Therapy. The three mini-books for learning the skill (the components) are scanned into Appendix B and are available for download from www.young-eisendrath.com. There are also multiple free teaching videos online for Real Dialogue. We won't review the three components of the skill here, except to remind you that they are specifically designed to (1) lower emotional threat levels from the beginning; (2) require stepping back from the reactivity of projective identification by requiring the parameters of speaking subjectively and listening mindfully; and (3) promote the development of a mindful gap between participants, permitting greater differentiation, respect, and creativity within the conversation.

The *method of Real Dialogue* is a co-facilitated conversation (although experienced facilitators may sometimes solo facilitate, using the four chairs as the solo Dialogue Therapist does). The physical set-up for RD is identical to the set-up for the co-therapy model of Dialogue Therapy (see, e.g., Figure 5.3a). The components of the method are trained currently as part of the DT training, but will in the future be bifurcated from the therapy training. Of course, mental health professionals who learn DT can also function as RD specialists. A person trained as an RD Specialist has completed the training and is certified as a specialist. The method is meant to be co-facilitated and it includes the following, adapted from DT (each of the following has been explained in detail in earlier chapters):

- Evaluation (opening conversation, interview, possibly Relational History)
- Six Questions (modified sometimes)
- Working on a Conflict (Coaching, Facilitating, Doubling/Alter-Ego, Unblocking, Reflecting Team)
- Wrap-Up
- Role Reversal (sometimes, depending on the situation)

In the Evaluation, the Real Dialogue co-facilitators enter the room with the participants, just as the co-therapists would in Dialogue Therapy. Participants are asked to sit in facing chairs.

The RD specialists may or may not know the details of the dispute being presented. If the situation involves an ongoing relationship (e.g., between team members, between adult child and parent, between co-workers or leaders on a team), the co-facilitators walk into the room, ask the participants to sit in the facing chairs, and the facilitators sit where the co-therapists sit in DT. Facilitators may begin with the prompt: "We would like to hear the two of you talk together about what you hope to get out of this meeting."

If the participants are strangers or barely know each other, then the meeting begins with each facilitator (who will team up with that partner) briefly interviewing that participant while the other participant sits in the "observer" seat as one does in Dialogue Therapy (see Figures 5.3 and b). The facilitator then says: "I would like to hear what you hope to get from this meeting." Then the facilitator uses the Real Dialogue skills to explore that topic until the participant says – "You've got it." The same interview then takes place with the other partner in the dialogue. When the desired outcomes are clear, the co-facilitators will speak together as a Reflecting Team in order to establish the aims of the conversation.

At this point, the facilitators will decide whether to use the Six Questions and the Relational History. If the relationship is ongoing for the dialogue partners, then the Six Questions may be used as they are or modified. When they are used, partners will talk briefly about some of their answers as they would in Dialogue Therapy. If the relationship is only momentary, then they are irrelevant. The same situation holds for the Relational History.

If partners have an ongoing relationship, then the Relational History may be relevant. If it is taken, then co-facilitators use the same setup and movement of chairs (see Figure 6.3a) that are used in Dialogue Therapy. If this is co-facilitation for ongoing relational partners (for example, married co-parents who are coming for a parenting conversation), then facilitators make the decision about what is useful from the Relational History Interview and make appropriate modifications.

If the Relational History is taken, then the main issues in their history should be summarized in the Wrap-Up – but *without a focus* on projective identification. Co-facilitation is not psychotherapy. Even though the co-facilitators may be therapists and may be helped by knowing the projective identifications, they will not be summarized in the Wrap-Up. In Real Dialogue, participants are not there for therapy or anything that seems like therapy (e.g., interpretation of their behaviors or history).

In setting up for Working on a Conflict (WOC), facilitators may formulate the conflict and/or the conflict may be formulated by participants, depending on the situation. The conflict is facilitated only for the outcomes of seeing, hearing, and feeling each other accurately, not for ongoing dynamics or clarifying projective identification. If partners are strangers, then the WOC session will be about a topic or conflict that has evolved out of their differences in some kind of work or family situation.

The objective of Real Dialogue is that each participant can clearly say (and be assessed to be accurate by the partner) and hear (as assessed by the partner) the other person's point of view, assumptions, and meanings. The methods used by co-facilitators will be Facilitating, Coaching, Doubling/Alter-Ego, Unblocking, and Reflecting Team, just as they are described for Dialogue Therapy, *except without any interpretations* of projection or projective identification. All interventions will focus on RD in terms of what participants are encouraged to say and hear, and in terms of how the facilitators speak to each other and with participants. Coaching, of course, may involve explaining and inquiring. Unblocking will certainly involve investigating what is going on and may involve trying to "get the bigger picture" of that individual's emotional meanings in the moment. Different from DT, the method of RD deals implicitly with the problems of projective identification, but not explicitly, although participants may become aware of their own projections or assumptions.

In the Wrap-Up at the end of each session, the co-facilitators summarize what has been accomplished and then ask for questions. Sometimes, partners find that they have more common ground than they thought. Sometimes, that is not the case. In any case, partners are encouraged to learn the skills of Real Dialogue to be used in emotionally intense or stressful conversations, although, as previously mentioned, they may not have learned them fully in the session(s). All of the resources for learning the skill will be made available to participants in the Wrap-Up – e.g., handouts, readings, website, videos, etc.

To summarize Real Dialogue's method, it uses the core skill of RD to explore the seen, heard, and felt experiences of each participant. Each facilitator works only with one participant over however many sessions are scheduled. That facilitator is both modeling and teaching the RD skill, but may also explore the narrative of the participant through a Relational History Interview and the Six Questions. Or, co-facilitators may decide *not* to use the Six Questions or the Relational History, but to work instead only within the methods for developing and enhancing the skill of RD in relation to the conflict at hand.

How long should sessions be and how many sessions should participants have? It depends. Everything is contextual in the method of Real Dialogue. Sometimes RD specialists are called into a business setting to deal with ongoing team members. Sometimes they are asked to facilitate a disagreement or to handle topics like anti-racism or vaccination when these topics are disrupting or occurring within a setting in which team members or leaders need to engage with, and understand, both sides of a dispute. If facilitators come into a setting as outsiders, then they must present to the group or organization a summary of what they plan to do with the RD sessions and how and when they plan to do it.

Often, Real Dialogue sessions are useful for other members in the setting to observe, so that the two sides of the conflict can be seen, heard, and felt by the entire community going through the experience. In working as consultants in an organizational setting (either live or on a live platform like Zoom), RD specialists will want to have a formal set-up that occurs in sessions that are at least two hours in duration and may recur over three or four meetings. This is because it takes some time and effort to set up the dialogue (i.e., go through the Evaluation and perhaps histories) between participants, just as in Dialogue Therapy.

However, when participants come *to* the Real Dialogue specialists for a consultation (in person or online), they may come only once. As we review the kinds of occasions and situations in which RD is useful, it will become evident that some people come only once because they want to talk respectfully about a stressful situation (e.g., a dispute between strangers about certain values), and not because they want to work together in an ongoing way. In a single intervention, co-facilitators typically will want at least two hours, and should even consider three hours. Less than two hours creates too much pressure when four adults are in the room and the atmosphere between participants is hostile.

How meetings are scheduled (their intervals and lengths), as well as what fee to charge, will depend on the co-facilitators' judgment and expertise. Real Dialogue can be considered a method of negotiation as well as a method of coaching and facilitation. Depending on the needs of clients, facilitators will tailor their approach. However, Real Dialogue specialists should be fully trained and certified, and should have completed their clinical consultations with certified Dialogue Therapists, per the requirements to complete the certification. But even when fully certified, we advise RD specialists to work with a co-facilitator who may be a Dialogue Therapist or another RD specialist. As in Dialogue Therapy, sessions in Real Dialogue are emotionally intense, challenging, and stressful. Having a co-facilitator is almost a requirement, even for expert facilitators. Why? Because of the projective identifications and all of their implied meanings, of course! In RD, facilitators are not interpreting the meanings, but they will feel them and they may "get" them.

Most of all, Real Dialogue facilitators must *not allow* participants to become hostile or to "fight it out" within sessions. Instead, from the start, as it is in Dialogue Therapy, facilitators will intervene to stop hostility and try to Coach or use Doubling with **you**-statements to prevent hostile rhetoric or objective claims (e.g., "*These are the facts.*"). If the participant still cannot Speak for Yourself or Listen Mindfully, after considerable intervention and Reflecting Team interaction with the co-facilitator, then Unblocking should be used. Unblocking allows RD specialists to control the session and compels the other participant to observe. This requires containment and builds capacity for objective empathy in the observer. And yet, this kind of "policing" of the participants entails a lot of emotional energy and thinking on one's feet. A co-facilitator is often the foundation of our confidence in being able to do what is required.

While Real Dialogue facilitation is a structured conversation in a co-facilitated set-up, it is clearly not psychotherapy, as we have already mentioned. Participants should be coming to learn how to work within an emotional space in order to see, hear, and feel each other during a difficult conversation. It is necessary for RD specialists to explain the realities of exactly what can be reasonably accomplished (e.g., mindful ways of speaking, listening, and Witnessing; increased differentiation and respect) and what cannot (e.g., resolution of conflicts, compromise, balance, or nonviolent communication) in marketing this method.

Sometimes clients and others may confuse the method with "conflict resolution." Or with "reconciliation." In fact, one of the *strengths* of Real Dialogue is that it aims only for differentiation and Witnessing, but not for compromise or solutions. We have discovered that people are more willing to enter into the process when they understand that it is not aimed at changing their views or opinions or frame of mind. All the same, these changes *might happen* as RD clears up the confusions, projections, and misapprehensions between the dialogue partners. While we call RD a form of negotiation (and it can be), it is also simply a form of mindfulness within conflict that permits more emotional space, lowering threat levels and increasing concentration, equanimity, and clarity of perception.

The practice of Real Dialogue

At the time of writing this, we are just beginning to develop (or dream about) a practice community for Real Dialogue. To be clear, in order to train as an RD Specialist (not a Dialogue Therapist), people are required *first* to learn the skill of RD. It can be learned online and will increasingly be available in video classes. Because it requires both an understanding of the snow globe of subjectivity, and some practice with guided meditation on one's own snow globe, learning the skill of RD is a prerequisite for training – if you are not training as a Dialogue Therapist. Putting all the RD skill training online is still a work in progress. Consequently, all RD specialists are now trained *within the training course for Dialogue Therapists*, learning alongside mental health professionals.

When Real Dialogue skill training is fully available online, we can begin to separate *training to become an RD specialist* from *training to become a Dialogue Therapist*. Ultimately, we hope to have all the RD method training online, through demo videos and live interactive online teaching. The RD teachers are now expert Dialogue Therapists, because there are not enough specialized RD facilitators yet to become teachers with backgrounds in business, education, activism, and so on, as described next.

The ultimate vision for Real Dialogue Skill and Method is to develop *practice communities* throughout the world, so that practitioners can become masters at facilitating RD in different kinds of settings. For example, we imagine a large community of RD for Co-Parenting, some of which could be dedicated to married parents, some to divorced or single parents, and so on. We also imagine a community of RD for Conversations About Death and Dying, which might be for family members and/or for religious organizations or hospice issues (e.g., how often and much morphine to give in the process of dying). Other communities might specialize in themes like RD for Leadership, RD for Collaborative Learning, RD for Divorce Mediation, RD for Executive Coaches, RD for Political Activism, RD for Anti-Racism, RD for Closing the Wealth Gap, and RD for Philanthropists. Our vision is a *worldwide movement of loosely affiliated* (but not incorporated) RD practitioners.

We also imagine an online magazine for *Real Dialogue: Ending Polarization and Respecting Conflict*. This magazine would allow RD practitioners, from various communities the world over, to share online and to help each other in their practices, with business development and also with tailoring the RD process to fit the particular needs of practice groups. In this way, we imagine that practitioners would develop the method over time so that it would become better suited to the needs of those caught in polarizations and repetitive conflicts. We imagine that the practice of RD, with its outreach and development through different practice communities and across different specialties, could potentially even help us to avoid wars. Practice groups could spring up where they are needed and be tailored to the special concerns of that group, although they would always include the skill and the method as designed – to contain emotional reactivity and commit to a mindful gap, differentiation, witnessing, and remaining curious.

There is one final practice community we feel seriously dedicated to developing: Real Dialogue for Family Estrangement. This would be a practice community dedicated to helping people learn to witness themselves and another from whom they have been painfully estranged. Again, the objective would not be reconciliation, but simply Witnessing. In *Fault Lines: Fractured Families and How to Mend Them*, sociologist Karl Pillemer (2020) presents his findings from nationwide research he conducted on family members who are estranged, and reports that at least 65 million Americans are estranged from a family member who is important to them; this is, he argues, an epidemic of estrangement, made worse by today's culture of polarized social and political differences in families. We envision a community of Real Dialogue for Family Estrangement that applies RD's particular strengths to help those who have experienced a deeply painful and shameful loss of family members due to estrangement.

Raising awareness for Real Dialogue skill, method, and practice

The vision of developing a worldwide online community of Real Dialogue practitioners seems a bit overwhelming, to us, at the moment. We are at the end of 2020 as we write this. All in-person Dialogue Therapy and RD training groups have been suspended until people are able to gather in person, in the US, and in Canada, where we have training groups. In the meantime, we are meeting online and trying to develop the tools needed to teach online. The vision for RD is strong and was in the process of getting support and funding when the virus shut it down, as it did to so many similar projects.

And yet, our original vision was also to develop online tools for Real Dialogue, as well as local organizations that can communicate, live and worldwide, through the online magazine, sharing their experiences and refinements of the method. It is still our fervent hope to teach the world about our vision for RD: about our subjective snow globes that require individual humility, mindfulness in speaking, listening during conflicts, and curiosity about others' points of view and perceptions. We have no doubt that RD, as a co-facilitated conversation, could end many hostilities with its apparently simple approach. We also have no doubt that there is little awareness, among ordinary people or societies and governments, of how projective identification inevitably leads to polarizations, especially when disputes and conflicts occur within the humiliation-rage cycle or result in dehumanizing others.

Dialogue Therapy for Couples has demonstrated over many decades that differentiation, Witnessing, and the practice of Real Dialogue allow even the most polarized and emotionally activated opponents – those who feel betrayed by their partner – the opportunity to see, hear, and feel each other with renewed curiosity. More important, RD used in the world at large would invite all of us to lower our emotional threat levels and open our ears to a new kind of *listening*, one that's imbued with concentration and equanimity, affording a new opportunity to see the world through our opponent's eyes, through which we would make deeper contact with our own humanity.

Bibliography

Hoffman, D. (2019). *The Case Against Reality: Why Evolution Hid the Truth from Our Eyes*. New York: W.W. Norton & Company, Inc.
Pillemer, K. (2020). *Fault Lines: Fractured Families and How to Mend Them*. New York: Avery.

Appendix A

Evaluation for Dialogue Therapy template

Evaluation

Intro for couple

I would like to hear the two of you talk to each other about why you are here. Please speak as though I were not here. You don't need to give me details because I will get those later through interviews. Just now, please speak with each other about your reasons for being here; you can speak in any way you want.

   NOTES (Use partners' initials. Get quotes as much as possible):

   (Use Unblocking if there is a lot of hostility or aggression. Face the aggressive person and say, "Please tell me what is going on for you right now." Otherwise, stay out of the conversation.)

Six Questions

I would like you to answer some questions in writing on the pad next to you. You can answer the questions in any way you want, taking as long as you want. You can use numbers, words, sentences, paragraphs or pictures. Some questions are easy to answer and some take more thought. This is a NOT a test. It is an assessment of how you feel today. Please put your first name in the corner of your paper. You will be able to take your answers home; these will not be secrets. Writing gives me/us a chance to hear from each of you individually. Please number your answers. You don't need to write the questions.

1   On a scale from 0–10, rate the value of this relationship for you person-ally where 0 means you could "take it or leave it" and 10 means it is "as valuable as oxygen, you couldn't live without it." Please give a number rating to the way you value this relationship, today.
2   From your perspective, what is the biggest problem or are the biggest problems in this relationship?
3   What are the greatest benefits of the relationship for you personally? What do you get from the relationship?

4   How do you think your partner (or your dialogue partner) rated the value of the relationship? How do you think they answered the first question?
5   How, in your opinion, did your partner answer the second question about problems in your relationship? What would your guess be?
6   How, in your view, did your partner answer the third question? What is your guess about what they see as the benefits of the relationship?

Collect the answers and scan them for what is most interesting/compelling/revealing for the partners to discuss.

Then: Please talk together about Questions #2 and #5, or #1 and #4, or #3 and #6.

(Again, do not intervene unless there is destructive hostility or aggression and then switch chairs and do some Unblocking.)

You may say: Please speak to each other, not to me. Ask questions of your partner and be sure you both understand the meanings of the words that you share.

NOTES on Six Questions and their discussion:

INTRO TO RELATIONAL HISTORY (Choose the partner you feel is more reactive, hurt, or aggressive.)

I would like to speak with XX first.

To begin:

I would like to review your sense of what the problem/problems are. (Summarize and paraphrase what you understand the person's answer to #2 and further conversation to mean.)

Then say: Please fill out this picture for me.

NOTES:

Make sure you understand the problems from that person's perspective. Use paraphrasing along the way.

RELATIONAL HISTORY: I am now going to do a review of this relationship and then other primary relationships in your life. We have about one hour for this task. I will structure the interview as we move along so that we can do this as effectively as possible. Your partner will be listening, but will not participate. Please don't turn around and ask your partner for answers to questions. I am most interested in exactly your point of view, your memory, your experiences. There are no "right" or "wrong" answers in this interview – only your answers. Does this make sense?

We are going to begin with how you met your partner. Please tell me how you met, your age then or the year, and the way you recall the circumstances.

NOTES:

How did you fall in love? When do you recall first feeling that you were attracted or wanted to be with this person? What happened next?

NOTES:

What about your first sexual experience? What do you recall? Who initiated it?

Milestones, going forward, NOTES:

How did you become a couple? Who pursued whom? Why?
Move in together?

Marriage proposal?
Wedding?
Children?
Betrayals?
Other issues?
Current living situation:
What is your age?
Your occupation?
Who lives with you at home now?
Anything else you want me to know?

NOTES (remember, try to get exact quotes):
Earlier marriages or live-in committed relationships?
In a nutshell, please tell me what attracted you to XX and why the relationship broke up.

The therapist should go backwards in time from most recent to earliest; make sure you get info on children from these relationships so that you know the details for step-families:
NOTES (Exact quotes when possible):

Most recent:
Next most recent:
Earliest:

Family of origin history

I will be asking you now about your family of origin. I will structure a couple of questions in an unusual sort of way. Please bear with me. I am trying to get outside of the stories you typically tell about your growing up, your most conscious or usual stories – because they won't help as much as the stories you don't know about. You can begin with either parent and I will ask you some questions and then we will fill out the history.

First parent

Please give me a picture of your parent. How did your mother/father look to you before you were ten years old? When you looked up to them, how did they look? Tall, short, old, young? Beautiful, shabby, appropriate, normal or something else?

Please give me a picture of your mother/father before you were ten years old:
NOTES:

Dress?
Personal Style?

Before ten, was this parent . . . affectionate (sit in lap, tuck you in, say "I love you" and comfort you)?

What do you recall about affection with your mother/father?

How about criticism or discipline before you were ten?

Anything else before ten?

Then how did things change after ten?

Was there conflict in your teenage years?

Bring me up to the present: what is your relationship with this parent like now?

Anything else you want me to know about your relationship with this parent?

Thanks. Now we are going to review your relationship with your other parent.

Please give me a picture of your other parent: how did your mother/father look to you before you were ten years old?

When you looked up to them, how did they look? Tall, short, old, young? Beautiful, shabby, appropriate, normal or something else?

Please give me a picture of your mother/father before you were ten years old:

NOTES:

Dress?

Personal Style?

Before ten, was this parent . . . affectionate (sit in lap, tuck you in, say "I love you" and comfort you)?

What do you recall about affection with your mother/father?

How about criticism or discipline before you were ten?

Anything else before ten?

Then how did things change after ten?

Was there conflict in your teenage years?

Bring me up to the present: what is your relationship with this parent like now?

Anything else you want me to know about your relationship with this parent?

How did you regard the relationship between your parents when you were young, before ten years old?

Later?

If there was a divorce or death, how did it affect you?

Was there a remarriage? Step-parents? Effects?

If there was a strife or conflict between your parents, did you line up with one side? How? Why?

Was there another parenting figure in your household growing up? Grandparent or aunt or uncle?

And how do you see your parents' relationship now?

And finally, I am going to ask a few questions about your siblings. Please give me the first name, age, and living situation of each sibling.

Name, age, relationship status, career

Sibling #1
Sibling #2
Sibling #3
Sibling #4

Others:
In brief, how do you relate to your siblings? Did you think/feel that one of them (or yourself) was a parent's favorite? Mother or father's favorite?

At the end of the empathy interview/Relational History

Summarize your hypothesis for yourself and give an overview to the client:

Look for phrases that overlap from one relationship/person to another:
Themes or dynamics that are repeated:
Your own notes to review each meeting:
To the client:

It seems to me that you have unconsciously or unwittingly invited your partner to play the part of your mother/father/sibling in your current relationship. It sounds like this part/or another part was played by your partner/spouse in your earlier relationship . . .

You get caught up in a triangle with your child/children/stepchild that plays out. . . .

Make sure your notes are clear on these themes. This will constitute a part of the projective identification

And now, you are going to switch chairs with your partner who will go through the same process.

To begin:
I would like to review your sense of what the problem/problems are. (Summarize and paraphrase what you understand the person's answer to #2 and further conversation to mean.)

Then say: Please fill out this picture for me.

NOTES:
Make sure you understand the problems from that person's perspective. Use paraphrasing along the way.

RELATIONAL HISTORY: I am now going to do a review of this relationship and then other primary relationships in your life. We have about one hour for this task. I will structure the interview as we move along so that we can do this as effectively as possible. Your partner will be listening, but will not participate. Please don't turn around and ask your partner for answers to questions. I am most interested in exactly your point of view, your memory, your experiences. There are no "right" or "wrong" answers in this interview – only your answers. Does this make sense?

We are going to begin with how you met your partner. Please tell me how you met, your age then or the year, and the way you recall the circumstances.
NOTES:

How did you fall in love? When do you recall first feeling that you were attracted or wanted to be with this person? What happened next?
NOTES:

What about your first sexual experience? What do you recall? Who initiated it?
Milestones, going forward, NOTES:

How did you become a couple? Who pursued whom? Why?
Move in together?
Marriage proposal?
Wedding?
Children?
Betrayals?
Other issues?
Current living situation:
What is your age?
Your occupation?
Who lives with you at home now?
Anything else you want me to know?

NOTES (remember, try to get exact quotes):
Earlier marriages or live-in committed relationships?
In a nutshell, please tell me what attracted you to XX and why the relationship broke up.

The therapist should go backwards in time from most recent to earliest; make sure you get info on children from these relationships so that you know the details for step-families:
NOTES (exact quotes when possible):

Most recent:
Next most recent:
Earliest:

Family of origin history

I will be asking you now about your family of origin. I will structure a couple of questions in an unusual sort of way. Please bear with me. I am trying to get outside of the stories you typically tell about your growing up, your most conscious or usual stories – because they won't help as much as the stories you don't know about. You can begin with either parent and I will ask you some questions and then we will fill out the history.

First parent

Please give me a picture of your parent. How did your mother/father look to you before you were ten years old? When you looked up to them, how did they look? Tall, short, old, young? Beautiful, shabby appropriate, normal or something else?

Please give me a picture of your mother/father before you were ten years old:

NOTES:

Dress?

Personal Style?

Before ten, was this parent . . . affectionate (sit in lap, tuck you in, say "I love you" and comfort you)?

What do you recall about affection with your mother/father?

How about criticism or discipline before you were ten?

Anything else before ten?

Then how did things change after ten?

Was there conflict in your teenage years?

Bring me up to the present: what is your relationship with this parent like now?

Anything else you want me to know about your relationship with this parent?

Thanks. Now we are going to review your relationship with your other parent.

Please give me a picture of your other parent: how did your mother/father look to you before you were ten years old?

When you looked up to them, how did they look? Tall, short, old, young? Beautiful, shabby, appropriate, normal or something else?

Please give me a picture of mother/father before you were ten years old:

NOTES:

Dress?

Personal Style?

Before ten, was this parent . . . affectionate (sit in lap, tuck you in, say "I love you" and comfort you)?

What do you recall about affection with your mother/father?

How about criticism or discipline before you were ten?

Anything else before ten?

Then how did things change after ten?

Was there conflict in your teenage years?

Bring me up to the present: what is your relationship with this parent like now?

Anything else you want me to know about your relationship with this parent?

How did you regard the relationship between your parents when you were young, before ten years old? Later?

If there was a divorce or death, how did it affect you?

Was there a remarriage? Step-parents? Effects?

If there was a strife or conflict between your parents, did you line up with one side? How? Why?

Was there another parenting figure in your household growing up? Grandparent or aunt or uncle?

And how do you see your parents' relationship now?

And finally, I am going to ask a few questions about your siblings. Please give me the first name, age, and living situation of each sibling.

Name, age, relationship status, career

Sibling #1
Sibling #2
Sibling #3
Sibling #4

Others:

In brief, how do you relate to your siblings? Did you think/feel that one of them (or yourself) was a parent's favorite? Mother or father's favorite?

At the end of the Relational History

Summarize your hypothesis for yourself and give an overview to the client:

Look for phrases that overlap from one relationship/person to another:

Themes or dynamics that are repeated:

Your own notes to review each meeting:

To the client:

It seems to me that you have unconsciously or unwittingly invited your partner to play the part of your mother/father/sibling in your current relationship. It sounds like this part/or another part was played by your partner/spouse in your earlier relationship . . .

You get caught up in a triangle with your child/children/stepchild that plays out. . . .

*MAKE SURE YOUR NOTES ARE CLEAR ON THESE
THEMES. THIS WILL CONSTITUTE YOUR RECORD OF
THE PARTNERS' PROJECTIVE IDENTIFICATION.*

WRAP-UP FOR BOTH PARTNERS AT END OF EVALUATION:

1   Statement of how you seem them playing out their internal theater together (projective identification):
2   Summary of the two "tribes" of their families and what is painful, disruptive, conflictual.
3   Most painful wounds/hurts. Active Aggression and Passive Aggression
4   Recommend/not recommend Dialogue Therapy
5   Reading assignments, primer
6   Set appointment for first or several session(s) of DT

First Session of DT:
NOTES:
I would like you to choose a conflict to work on in this session.

Second Session of DT:
Third Session of DT:
Subsequent Sessions of DT:
Wrap-Up at Conclusion of DT:
NOTES about any concerns on ending:
Date for six-months follow-up:
NOTES FROM SIX-MONTHS FOLLOW-UP:
NOTES FROM ANY FURTHER SESSIONS:

Appendix B

Section 1

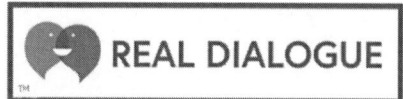

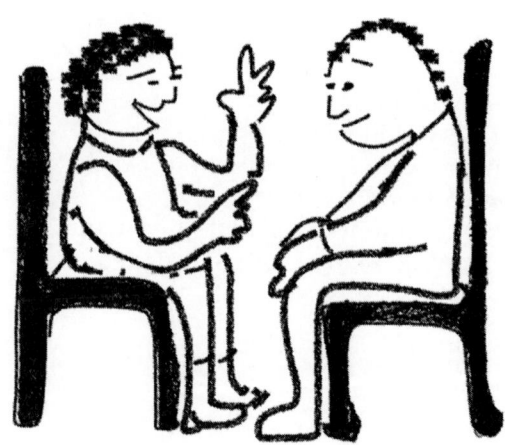

Real Dialogue
The Skill: Volume 1
Speaking for Yourself

Polly Young-Eisendrath, Ph.D.

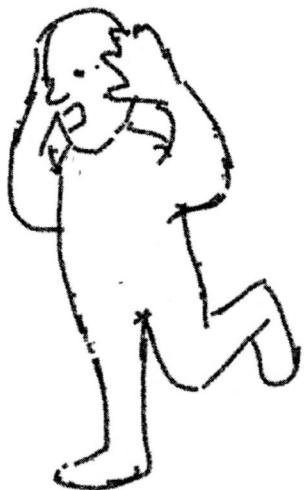

Do you sometimes feel like you want to run out of the
room or just scream when you've repeatedly said the
same thing, clearly and slowly, to someone you want
to influence (maybe someone you're supposed to love
or believe in) and they JUST DON'T GET IT???

You need the skill of Real Dialogue to help
you maintain a mindful space for give and take

 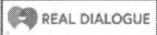

during times of emotional threat, stress, and perceived offense.

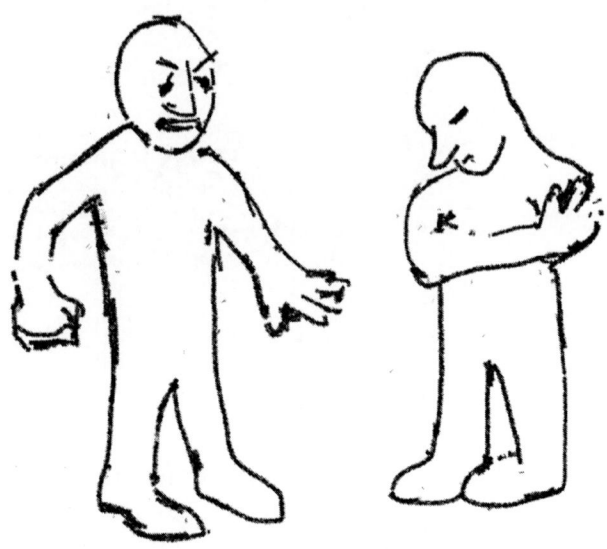

Real Dialogue is a skill that comes originally from Dialogue Therapy, developed to help couples deal with repetitive conflicts.

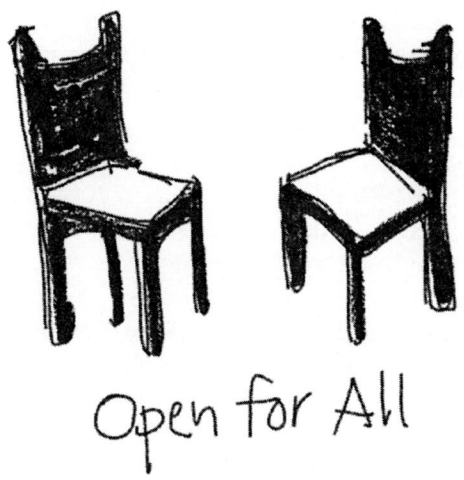

Open for All

Now it is available to all to use in negotiations and conflicts of opposing sides.

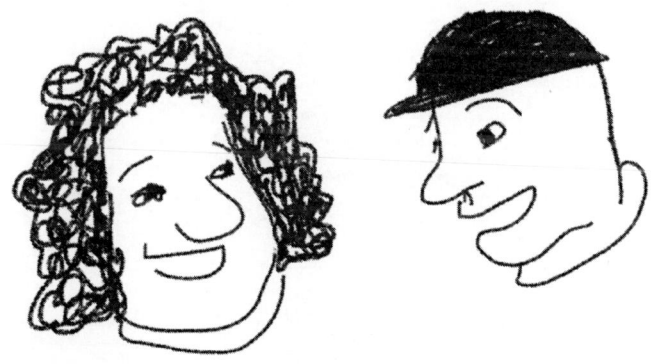

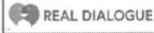

Real Dialogue counteracts our natural tendencies to defend ourselves by habitually avoiding conflict or dehumanizing someone else.

Real Dialogue gives us an alternative to feeling unseen and unknown when we are in states of conflict, emotional agitation, deep disagreement, or irritation. Through it, we can reach lasting solutions to our problems by drawing on both sides and making new discoveries, even WHILE STILL DISAGREEING. Our conflicts become useful.

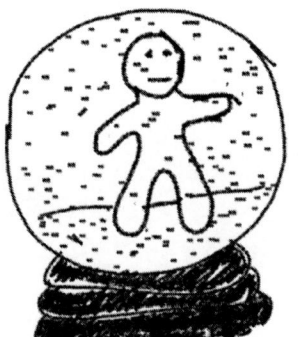

Snow globe of Being Human

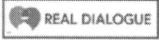

Real Dialogue allows people on different sides, each with legitimate perceptions and authentic points of view, to find a mindful space even if they profoundly disagree and are in emotional pain.

Maybe you are wondering:

"WHY, WHY, WHY do good people get into such hateful polarizations?? Why do family members, co-workers, and partners scape-goat each other and create enemies? WHAT IS WRONG?"

EACH OF US IS TRAPPED IN A SNOW GLOBE! Because we are each in our own snow globe of subjectivity we see, hear, and feel things VERY differently. When you have two people, you have two WORLDS.

Especially when we feel emotionally threatened because someone who is important to us, or someone who has power over us, JUST DOESN'T GET WHAT WE MEAN: our snow globe gets shaken up and we pay attention to the storm inside. In place of listening, we start rehearsing our own speeches. We can't seem to tolerate what the other person is saying and that's when the storm inside overtakes our eyes, our ears, and our not-ever-very-accurate ability to witness.

Instead, Real Dialogue teaches us that we have to
S-L-O-W DOWN ALL OF OUR FACULTIES so that we
can speak for ourselves (modestly, subjectively, not
shaming/blaming) and check on what we have heard
from the other person to see if we have listened to

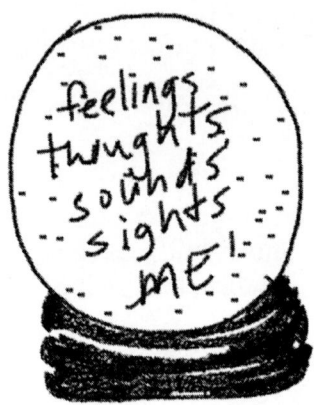

anything other than the voice in our own head.

Instead of slowing down, though, we naturally speed
up to defend our own reality. Of course we do, because
the stakes are high when we are in a conflict with someone who is important to us.

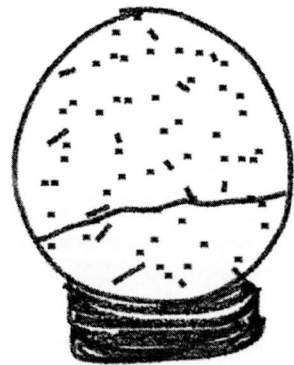

Real Dialogue teaches us first about our subjective life
and its complex snow globe of six competing realities:

1. Hearing Out (sounds and voices outside body)
2. Hearing In (sounds and voices inside our head)
3. Seeing Out (images and colors and light outside)
4. Seeing In (images and colors in the mind's eye)
5. Feeling Out (sensations of body and surroundings)
6. Feeling In (sensations of emotions in body)

Each human snow globe is a busy place especially
when it needs defending, protecting, or promoting.

 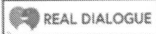

When two snow globes are shaken up and each human is trying to respond "objectively" and to "find the truth of the matter," there will be a fierce and dangerous tangle of subjectivities.

To begin disentangling, the First Rule of Real Dialogue is "speak for yourself." This means much more than using "I-statements." It means recognizing that you are in your OWN snow globe and NO ONE outside "makes you feel" the way you feel, unless they are physically harming you. There are some rigid perceptual and emotional habits in your snow globe that were laid down to protect you in your early life. You respond by old habits when you feel threatened. No one else is making that happen.

Real Dialogue requires that you vow to speak for yourself subjectively — such as "It's my impression, my opinion, my memory..." and stay away from ANY objective statements such as "It was July 3rd when" or "Your mother called us before..." or "The facts are" or many other statements that derail the issues being talked about and take us into endless searches for "evidence" about who is "right" and who is "wrong." With few exceptions (you were videotaped?) the evidence does not exist.

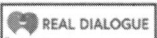

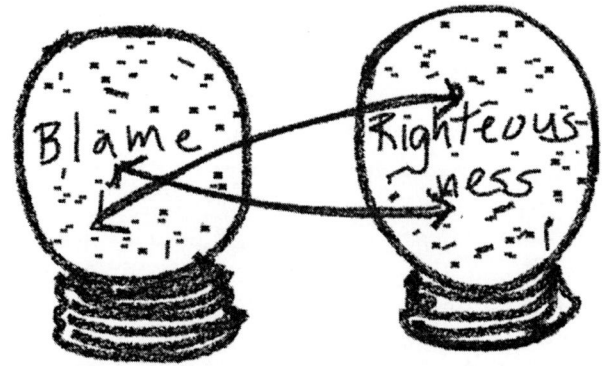

What you are faced with instead is two snow globes that are badly shaken up. Typically, there are no helpful facts, except that two snow globes need to get back into communication if their problem, conflict, dispute, need, plan, predicament, mistake or emergency is going to get solved.

Making things more complicated is the humiliation-rage cycle which gets going because one or both people feel they have been faulted or blamed in a humiliating way. They have the emotional experience of "being exposed" and that evokes RAGE. Rage may be expressed by walking away and stonewalling, refusing to speak or it may be expressed through explosions of aggression and threats that may be directed at the other person, physical objects around them, or at oneself (e.g. hitting one's own head or

REAL DIALOGUE

Our lack of consensus only increases when we are emotionally jarred. Our highly subjective "reality" makes us VERY poor eye witnesses. We are unable to agree about what is actually happening much of the time. That's why we argue so much about "what is true" or "what the facts are."

But that doesn't mean you are unaffected by what others say, feel and otherwise express. When someone expresses emotion in a bold or obvious way, you are definitely affected. Emotion that is expressed evokes emotions. Because you are in your own subjective snow globe, though, you cannot know exactly what is evoked in someone else and they cannot know your emotions for certain either, without asking you.

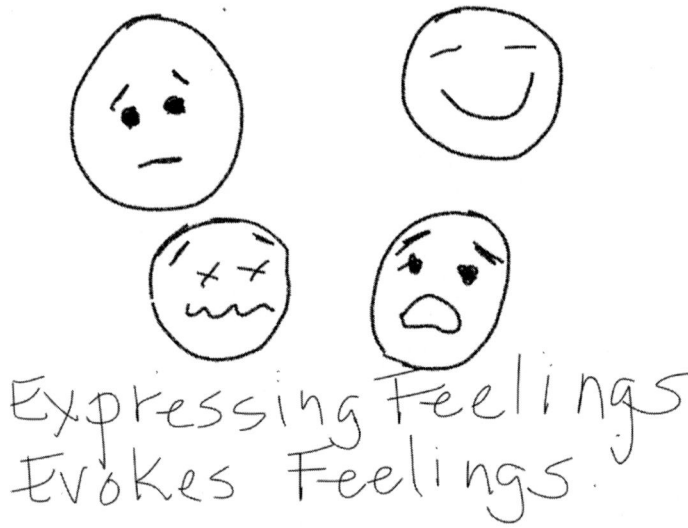

Expressing Feelings Evokes Feelings.

Here are some typical you-statements (and their implied meanings) that evoke rage during conflict, stated rhetorically as "Don't you even care?":

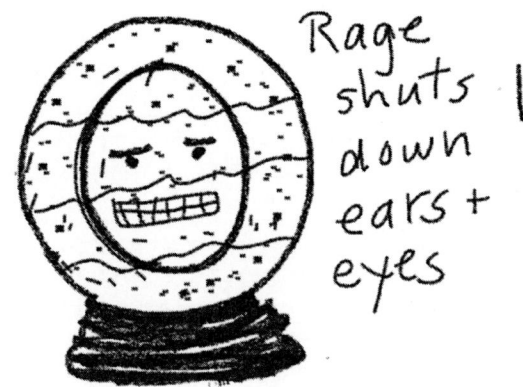

Rage shuts down ears + eyes

Don't you care about ...		(And so, you are...)
OUR CHILDREN	=	bad parent
CLIMATE CHANGE	=	climate denier
OUTCOMES	=	stupid or self-centered
SCIENCE	=	stupid, uninformed
RACISM	=	racist
SEXISM	=	sexist
WHETHER I AM HAPPY	=	narcissist
CARING FOR OTHERS	=	narcissist
KNOWING ABOUT ME	=	narcissist

REAL DIALOGUE

The speaker thinks the above statements are "just giving you my opinion" but the attack on the other person is harsh and implied, evoking rage in the face of the humiliation.

Other kinds of destructive you-statements are sneaked in as if they are statements of "feelings":
"I feel manipulated by you"
"I feel afraid to speak to you"
"I feel like you should...(exercise, sleep)...more"
"I feel you are not interested in what I say"

Even though these statements are not saying "You are self-centered, ill-informed or unmotivated," they imply it. These shaming implications evoke rage and in most cases the other person will either attack, defend, stonewall or humiliate back.

Most of us know that we have a "limbic system," the middle part of a brain, sitting right behind our eyes and the frontal cortex; it contains one small almond-shaped organ called the amygdala. That organ activates the flight-fight-freeze respond to THREAT. The amygdala is a kind of crude system: easy to activate and hard to de-activate.

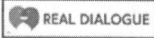

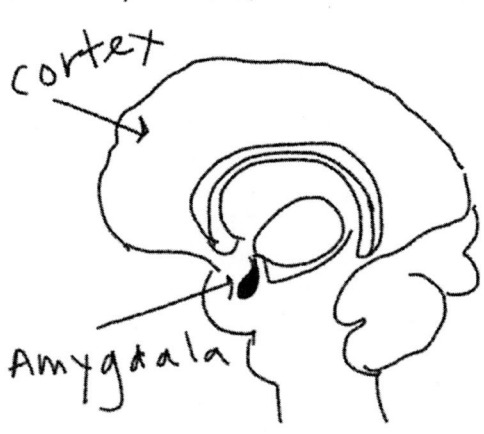

Profile of human brain

cortex

Amygdala

We humans are very sensitive to our social status (group ranking) because we usually hang around in groups called families, organizations, corporations, societies, nations. Within these groups we are all self-promoting and self-protective. If we feel emotionally threatened in the group, we will react with the flight-fight-freeze response. Feeling HUMILIATED means that you feel your status is reduced and/or your flaws and weaknesses are exposed.

For humans enclosed in their snow globes humiliation evokes rage – a hopeless and sometimes uncontrollable violence and self-protection.

IN REAL DIALOGUE you AVOID EMOTIONAL THREATS that evoke the rage response. That means you avoid saying or implying something that is humiliating or shaming or suggests that other person is of a lower status, toxic or disgusting.

When you begin a Real Dialogue with someone with whom you are in conflict and with whom you must negotiate, especially if it seems that person is "wrong" or misperceives you, NEVER begin with a litany of faults such as:

You never...
You always...
You don't follow through...
You might be amazing, but...
because you want to avoid enraging that person from the start.

You recognize that you are enclosed in your own snow globe. You speak with modesty from your own perspective and you are curious to understand the other's perspective, even if you totally disagree or feel hurt by it.

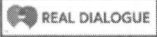

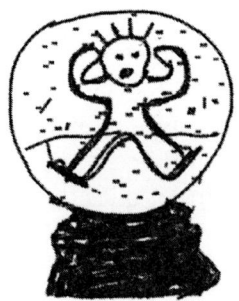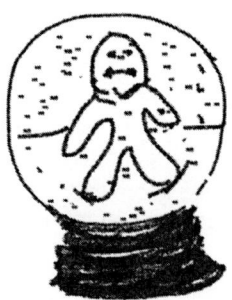

Here are some good openers for Real Dialogue:

Help me understand what you mean by...

I want to work out our differences and I would like to know why you said that to me.

You and I are working on this project together and I want to finish it well. Help me see your point of view more clearly...

I am feeling hurt and angry about what I believe you said to me and I would like to repair my trust in you. Can I give you my impression of what I heard you say to me?

I would like to hear from you about what you are experiencing right now.

 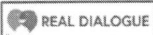

By avoiding implied or direct accusations of the other person as though the other person has caused your pain, suffering, humiliation, or anxiety, it is important to begin on the best foot possible.

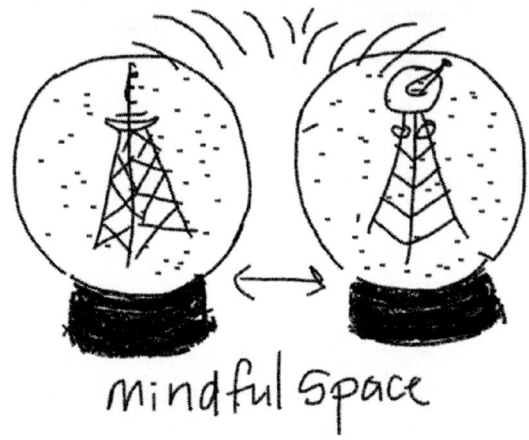

mindful space

As you move along in the conversation, you stick with the modesty of your snow globe and you gradually build a radio tower signal base in your snow globe that can pick up the messages from the other snow globe in a way that makes communication work:

"This is the way I remember it..."
"Here is my impression..."
"I would like our conversation to take this direction, how about you?"

"I have some negative feelings about something I believe you said and that is why I have hesitated to trust you. I want to be sure I didn't misunderstand what you are saying."

During a Real Dialogue you appreciate the space between your snow globe and the other person's. You enjoy the fact that you are, in fact, two different worlds and that many new ideas, perspectives, experiences can be discovered if you can open the communication between you and keep it open during the most painful and agitating differences. You also recognize that what you "observe" in another is coming from your perspective in your own snow globe colored by your emotional habits and defenses.

Speaking for Yourself is an application of mindfulness practice: you pay close attention to your own experience, you accept your experience as tolerable, and you find a way to speak your truth without blaming someone for it. If you cannot do this with a particular person because you only want to blame or humiliate them, then you break off the communication because it will lead only to destructiveness.

As you learn more and more about the skill of Speaking for Yourself, you feel more confident in going through conflicts and negotiations. You learn how to avoid the humiliation-rage cycle. You know how to stay away from fight or flight reactivity. You begin to enjoy saying things subjectively, modestly, and you even begin to wonder what is "objective" — outside of mathematics, data analysis, and some computation (and even then there can be different interpretations).

Learning how to Speak for Yourself means that you don't have to walk away from talking about painful and divisive topics. You can, of course, draw a boundary if you find that another person refuses a real dialogue and attacks or harms you in a way that you cannot respond to.

Largely, though, you come to appreciate and embrace personal conflicts because we need them in order to change our minds. As the Canadian singer-songwriter Leonard Cohen says in his ballad "Different Sides":

"We find ourselves on different sides of a line nobody drew.

"While it might be One in the Higher Eye, down here where we live it is Two."

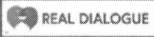

In our next primer on Real Dialogue, we will examine the issues involved with keeping your ears open during painful conflict through Paraphrasing or Mindful Listening.

The Skill: Volume 1

REAL DIALOGUE

Section 2

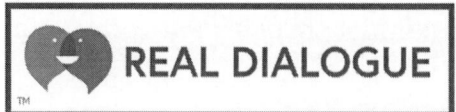

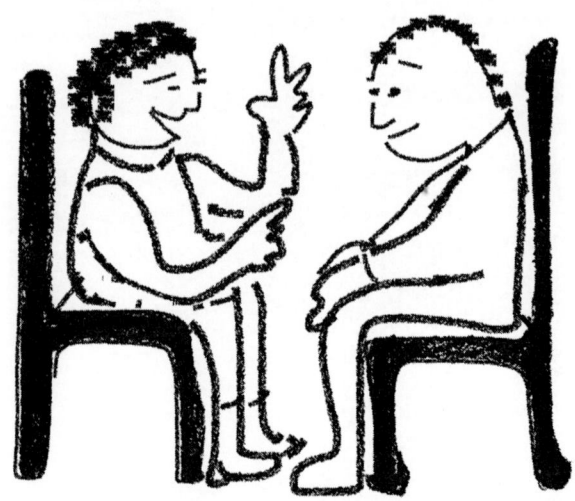

Real Dialogue
The Skill: Volume 2
Mindful Listening: Paraphrasing

Polly Young-Eisendrath, Ph.D.

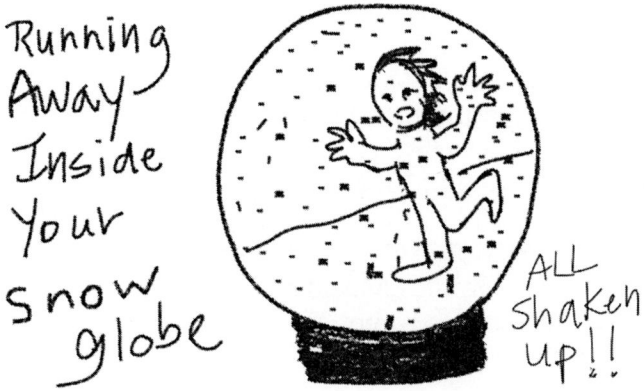

We have already learned the First Rule of Real Dialogue, Speaking for Yourself. Now we are ready to get to the HARD part — yes, the listening part.

Remember that we are all stuck inside of our own snow globes of subjectivity in which we have a confusing mix of seeing, hearing, and feeling that makes it hard to witness what is going on inside of someone else's snow globe or even to care.

REAL DIALOGUE

When we are faced with difficult conversations that kick us into self-protection and self-promotion, we get confused about how to listen, why to listen, and what to listen to. Sometimes we just give up trying. Mostly we react in the fight-flight mode and only listen to what we are saying INSIDE OUR OWN HEADS.

WHAT'S A DIFFICULT CONVERSATION? Anything that stirs up our self-promoting and self-protecting responses...could be an emotional threat from someone we love, an opinion or idea that we totally disagree with, a criticism that seems humiliating, or even someone's tone of voice that sounds urgent.

Difficult conversations are made worse by the need to make a decision, a plan, deal with an emergency, or work with the other person on a big project that goes on over a long time. These factors add STRESS. Often people who emotionally activate each other and have to make decisions, plans, or deal with work projects just give up. They are afraid of engaging in conflicts, or becoming enraged, because they feel humiliated by not seeming to be able to get their ideas across or to solve problems together.

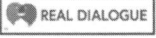

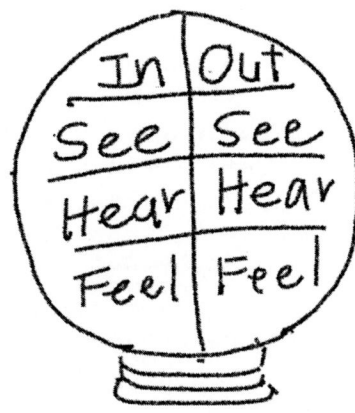

Difficult conversations stir up the fight-flight response that shakes up our snow globes making it very hard for us to handle our own perceptions because of the confusion about what we are seeing, hearing, feeling.

Let's review the six aspects of our subjectivity and the confusing ways in which we see, hear, feel others and the world around us. No matter the situation, whether we are shaken up or not, we are not simply seeing and hearing "things" as they are.

Instead, we mix up our perceptions (inside/outside) in a way that makes stepping into another's shoes or "really listening" very difficult:

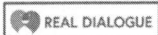

Seeing In/Out: We see "out in the world" including others, but we also see "into the mind's eye" in images, pictures, colors. We can make serious mistakes because the mind's eye can cause us to "perceive" something like another person having a threatening look when it's not happening. We don't see each other clearly, but rather perceive each other through the "glass darkly" of our own snow globes.

Hearing In/Out: It seems as though we have even more trouble hearing another person when we are activated emotionally.

Unconsciously and automatically we close up our ears. We don't want to hear something that activates that old amygdala or associates with something threatening. Instead of L I S T E N I N G we turn up the volume of talking to ourselves and rehearse what we are about to say or simply start screaming inside to ourselves.

As you practice the skill of Mindful Listening, you might be surprised at how little you actually hear when you are listening while being emotionally activated.

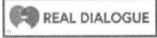

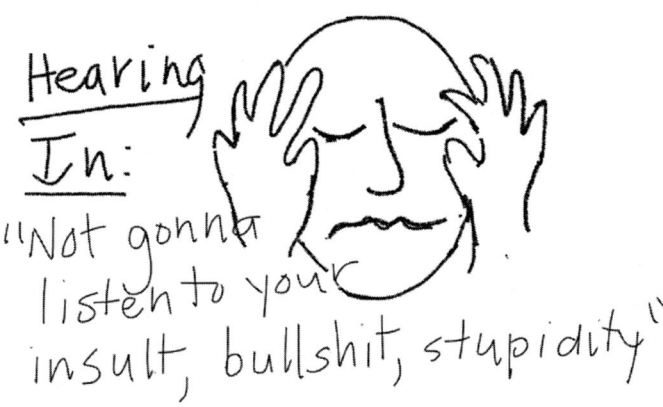

Hearing
In:
"Not gonna listen to your insult, bullshit, stupidity"

Feeling In/Out : The term "feeling" here applies to both physical sensations of what our bodies are experiencing (aches, pains, pleasures, energy) and the ways our emotions (activating or motivating systems) convey subjective meaning and trigger what is called *emotional memory* (neural reaction that causes us to feel right NOW precisely like we felt in the past, even if we don't have any memory of that earlier event).

All of these aspects of feeling often contribute to our being mistaken about what is happening in the present moment. When we feel "upset" or "angry" or "sad" or other "negative" emotional states, we are distressed in ways that range from mild to extreme. In these states,

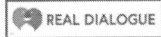 REAL DIALOGUE

we may feel "triggered" or "unsafe." Then we may become especially self-protective and/or self-promoting ("I feel traumatized and I am going to STAND up for MY rights!"). Our painful emotional states are being produced inside our own snow globe and may or may

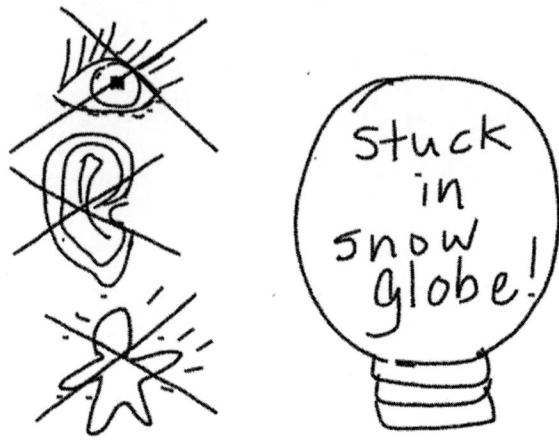

not be relevant to the what the other person is doing or saying. The way we are perceiving the other person is SUBJECTIVE from inside our own snow globe.

Unfortunately, and sadly, we may have NO ability to see, hear, feel the other's subjectivity when our own snow globe is shaken up. We are as far away from "being objective" as we can be.

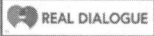

This is not a place from which we should begin a
negotiation, make an accusation, or decide to quit/
separate/leave/fire the other person.

Instead we need to develop Mindful Listening as a tool
for Real Dialogue; this gives us the opportunity to find
out about what is going on in the other person's
snow globe.

Mindful Listening is the capacity to step back
from our subjective shake-up into a more matter-of-

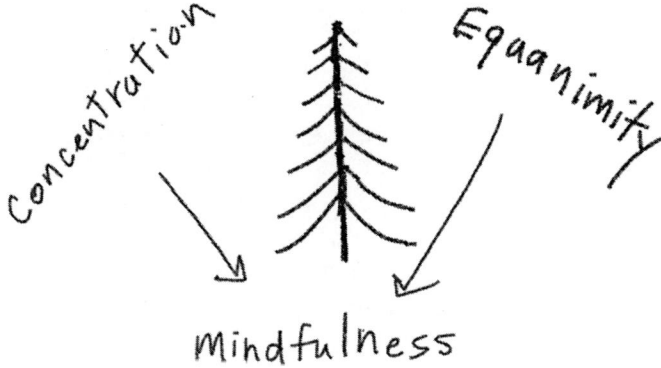

fact state of mind in which we may be able to open our
ears, eyes, and feelings to even the most painful ideas
and thoughts that someone is trying to convey to us.

What is Mindfulness??

You have probably heard a LOT about Mindfulness
and you may be confused about what it is and whether
it makes sense to ordinary distracted people (like you
or me).

Mindfulness is a certain kind of awareness that we
can cultivate or develop by exercising our
"mindfulness muscles." Those muscles can be
exercised through meditation and/or through
Speaking for Yourself and Mindful Listening in Real
Dialogue.

Mindfulness combines two states of being:
concentration and equanimity. Together they increase
mental clarity; they allow us to see, hear, feel with
greater openness to our whole experience.

Concentration supports our awareness with alertness
and an awakened attitude; it's like the trunk of the
pine tree which is straight and strong. Equanimity, like
the branches of the pine tree, permits us to just hang
out or relax with our experiences. Concentration allows
us to remember and be alert. Equanimity provides us
with a gentle matter-of-fact attitude, no matter how
painful or distressing the experience is.

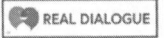

Together, these two states permit us to pay close attention to what is actually happening without trying to push (fight) or pull back (flee) on our experience.

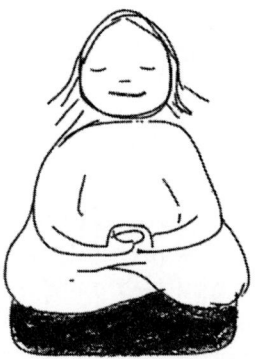

Applying Mindfulness to your skillful listening during a difficult conversation will develop your Mindfulness muscles or strengthen them if you already have them. Often people develop Mindfulness only in solitary or group situations — meditating as an individual or getting guidance in a group.

Almost never do people learn how to meditate in the middle of a difficult conversation! And yet, we need

 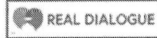

Mindfulness skills primarily when we are emotionally activated. When we are not activated, we may naturally cultivate enough concentration and equanimity to get around in life. Of course, we develop concentration and equanimity in our meditation practice but that won't translate directly to listening accurately in difficult conversations.

Many people may even be confused about WHY they should meditate. We should NOT meditate pimarily to get better at meditating. We should meditate to get better at life or living. Meditation is not primarily for calming down (a massage is probably better for that). Meditation should help us develop our mindfulness muscles so that we can use them when we are walking around and relating to others.

What better way to use our Mindfulness muscles than in difficult conversations with family members, team members at work, and those we plan and deliberate with in our communities and societies?

In these challenging and precious situations we need to be able to open our eyes, ears, and emotions to include another's subjectivity and work with BOTH sides of an issue so that we can find the creative, mutual outcomes and discoveries that we all want.

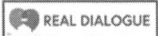

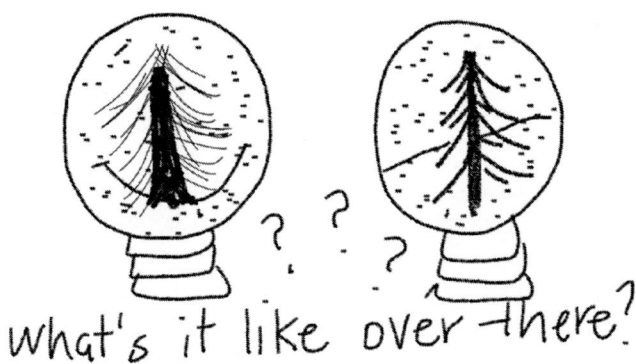

In Real Dialogue, we cultivate the tools of Mindful Listening by applying "paraphrasing" in a new and important way.

Instead of parroting or repeating back "Here's what I heard you say..." we develop the skill of listening deeply to the other's experience and then looking through our mind's eye to SEE if we can perceive their point of view, the view from their snow globe. In seeing another's point of view, we are not AGREEING or COMPROMISING unless we want to. Agreement or compromise is not the point.

The point is to develop a Mindful Gap in which you can know each other through your differences. Of

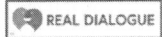

course, you might discover that you don't disagree as much as you initially thought and so you can skillfully maneuver through the conflict, and clarify yourself just through Speaking for Yourself and Mindful Listening.

Listening in this way allows you to step into the other's snow globe and see what it's like. Then you check out your perception by saying to the other person "Here's the way I am understanding what you are saying." You choose words that mirror or deepen the other person's language and assumptions without parroting them. You learn to be careful to eliminate hidden zingers that come from your snow globe.

When you are finished, you check: "Did I get that?" And "Is there more?" The paraphrasing is complete only at the point when the other person says "You really got it!" At that moment there will be a palpable relief for both people – the one speaking and the one listening.

Paraphrasing or Mindful Listening is necessary at times of emotional agitation or painful differences. Many times in Mindful Listening and paraphrasing, we have to go back to the drawing board because of our own subjective experience has disrupted our ability to see/hear/feel what the other is saying. Only when the other person agrees that we understand do we get the green light to "go ahead."

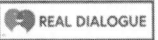

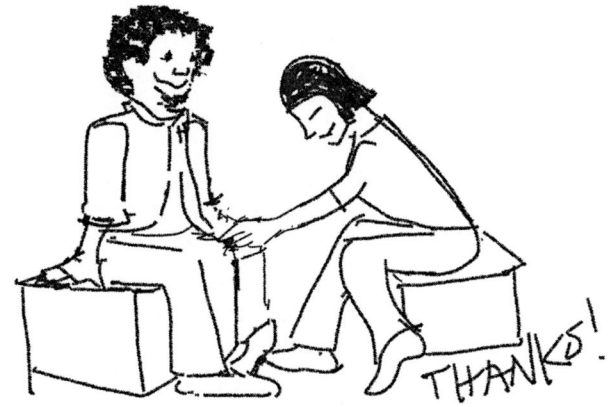

When we have understood the other person, there is a wonderful relief, gratitude and even joy. When Mindful Listening goes both ways, then two people remove the obstacles to having creative and fruitful conflicts.

Speaking for Yourself, Listening Mindfully, and Remaining Curious are the three components of the skill of Real Dialogue. You develop the skill to use anywhere. If you have a friend, partner, grown child, sibling, co-worker, or associate who can practice it with you, you will have an especially good chance of feeling the deep relief of its benefits. But even if you simply practice the skill yourself, you will find

 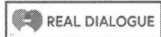

yourself more confident, open-minded, and curious in even the most distressing conflicts.

People do not have to agree or compromise to have fruitful conflicts or disagreements. (Obviously, this is not the same thing as "agreeing to disagree" which is simply the avoidance of exploring a topic.)

As soon as you begin to feel confident that you can speak for yourself and listen mindfully, then you know that you will never have to agree falsely in order to work together on the challenges that face you. You can use the skill of Real Dialogue to get through the weeds of conversation so that you can return to the garden of understanding and working together.

And yet, it's not as though Real Dialogue is ever a done-deal. It's always a work in progress. You have to apply your skills each time that your snow globe is shaken. Like any other practice — playing tennis, playing the piano, meditating — when you get good at Real Dialogue, you will want to engage in creating ever more open mindful space between your snow globe and another's. You will also find you want to apply Real Dialogue in different aspects of your life – at home, at work, and in the world.

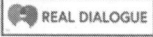

In the final volume we will take up the third skill of Real Dialogue: Remaining Curious. This is the challenge to remain engaged and interested about others' snow globe even when you think you "already know" you believe something the opposite side of what is being said.

REAL DIALOGUE

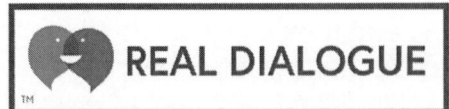

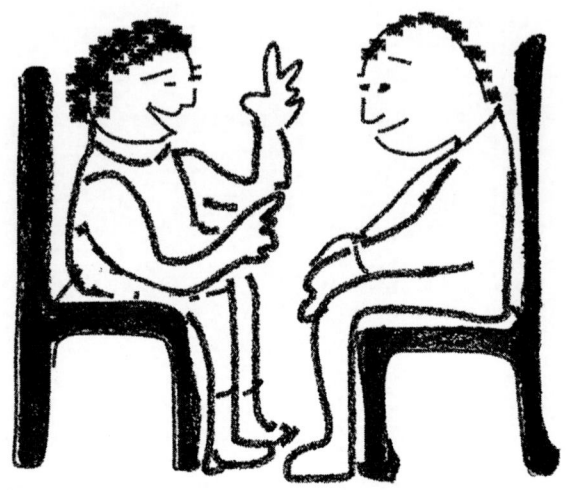

Real Dialogue
The Skill: Volume 3
Remaining Curious

Polly Young-Eisendrath, Ph.D.

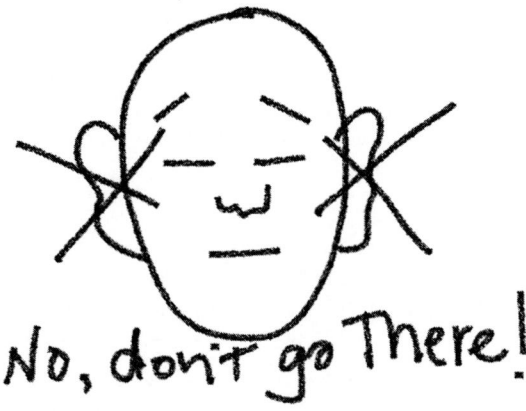

If you want to keep a lively and engaged feeling about your life, you must remain curious about what you hear and see. This vital connection to moment-to-moment reality can mean the difference between feeling happy and creative or irritated and confused, especially in relating to others.

And yet, if someone you know well, your partner or friend or coworker, begins talking about a topic and you believe you "have heard it all before," you might find yourself saying "OH NO, I know where THIS is going!" and you close your ears.

Or, you are talking with someone about a topic that hits a nerve, especially an opinionated nerve, and you find yourself saying "I know where THIS is going and I don't want to go there!" Instead of mindfully l-i-s-t-e-n-i-n-g to what the other person is saying, you shut down your curiosity.

 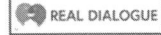

What's happening? You are hearing the voices
(HEARING IN) in your own head. You are HEARING IN
and not HEARING OUT. You are listening to yourself.
You may be talking to yourself about the waste of time
this will be or about how reactive you will become or
how predictable this person is who "always gets into"
this topic.

Inside your own snow globe, you have little to no
interest in what the other person is saying. Instead
of using your ears to HEAR OUT and listen to what
the other person is saying, you are HEARING IN to
yourself speaking in the same old ways. No wonder this
encounter is tedious. You are saying the same blahblah-
blah to yourself that you always say.

And you may also say something emotionally
threatening to the other person, like "Hey, I don't want
to go into THIS again!" Or, something humiliating, like
"I have heard ALL THIS BEFORE!" Then, suddenly, the
two of you are in the humiliation-rage cycle. Naturally,
your encounter becomes the SAME OLD fight-flight
reactivity you had wanted to avoid.

YOU are directing what's going on in your own snow
globe. You are rehearsing the same old script in your
own head and listening to yourself in your own ears. It's
deadening and repetitive. It's not the other person who
is saying "the same old thing," it's YOU!

Perhaps you have asked yourself this question: Is it
possible to remain curious about someone you have
known for a long time? Or about someone whom you

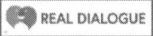

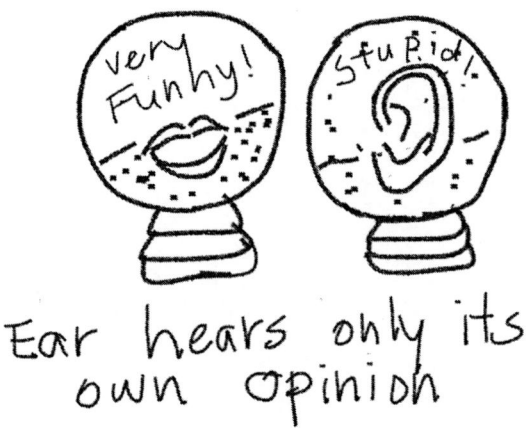

don't especially like? Or about a family member or
co-worker who pushes your buttons? Is it possible to
remain engaged in an interesting conversation with
another person who holds an opinion that you do not
agree with? The answer to all of these questions is
YES, it is. And your life/world will become more
interesting if you learn how to do this. Then, you can
interact with the truth – that EVERYTHING CHANGES
moment-to-moment.

The reality of impermanence will get gradually clarified
inside your own snow globe! Instead of the same old
blah-blah in your snow globe or that same rigid little
dance you have always done, you will start receiving
more contact through your ears, eyes, and body
sensations with the changing reality within and
outside of you.

In this volume of Real Dialogue you will learn how to
remain curious during times of emotional threats,
repetitive conflicts and difficult conversations by

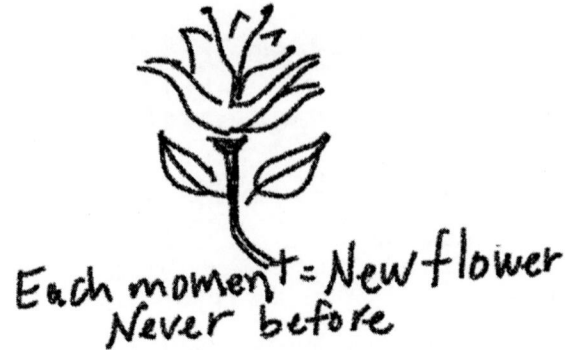

Each moment = New flower
Never before

applying the first two rules of Real Dialogue – Speaking for Yourself and Listening Mindfully – within the larger sense of the "Don't Know Mind." The Don't Know Mind means the experience of being in the present moment of freshly seeing/hearing/feeling things.

In order to hold this fresh connection to seeing/hearing/feeling in your own snow globe, you need first to embrace the fact that everything (including you) changes from moment to moment: this is the reality of Impermanence. You may say "OK, I know we are always only in the NOW and the present moment fades rapidly. STILL, I have heard my partner tell that joke a thousand times and it's always the same joke!"

The joke is not "always the same" inside your partner's snow globe; in fact, your partner is telling it in a particular moment because it is MEANINGFUL in a whole new way. Your partner is telling the joke because it seems really funny in this moment.

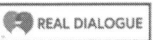 REAL DIALOGUE   The Skill: Volume 3   5

The most widely quoted line in Leonard Cohen's beloved song *Anthem* is "There's a crack in everything, and that's how the light gets in." I want to re-write that line to say "There's a GAP between everyone and that's how the LOVE gets in."Holding a Mindful Gap between your ears Hearing In and Hearing Out, you can remain OPEN

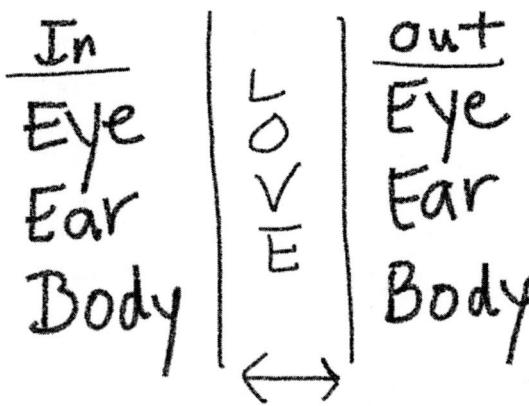

to hearing the other person in a whole new way. The first principle of Remaining Curious is to recognize that each moment is new and fresh, and if you are having "the same old experience" it is YOU who is manufacturing it.

If you REALLY know that there is no "same old stuff" (even the stuff you rehearse in your own mind changes with the circumstances you are in) then each new

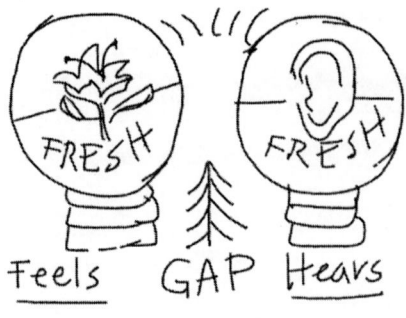

situation, each moment, each joke is engaging and fresh. You are hearing it for the first time in these circumstances.

You might even find your own blah-blah interesting, funny, sad, or stupid in a whole NEW way.

The second rule to Remaining Curious is "MIND the GAP!!" Keep a not-knowing gap between your snow globe and another's, especially when you believe you have "heard all this before!!"

You may have heard the Zen phrase "Don't-Know Mind." This is the mind that sees/hears/feels freshly in every moment. This is the mind that doesn't know IN ADVANCE exactly what something means. This is the mind you cultivate in Real Dialogue.

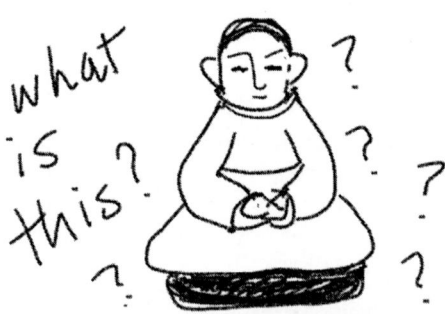

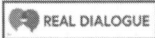

Too often we apply fresh awareness only when we are calm or at peace. OH! new flower, new scent, new spring in my step, new panorama, new phrasing of the joke, new telling of her story. Remaining Curious in Real Dialogue means that you apply the Don't-Know Mind when you are agitated and thrown, especially in those emotionally charged and vexing conversations that tend to throw you again and again.

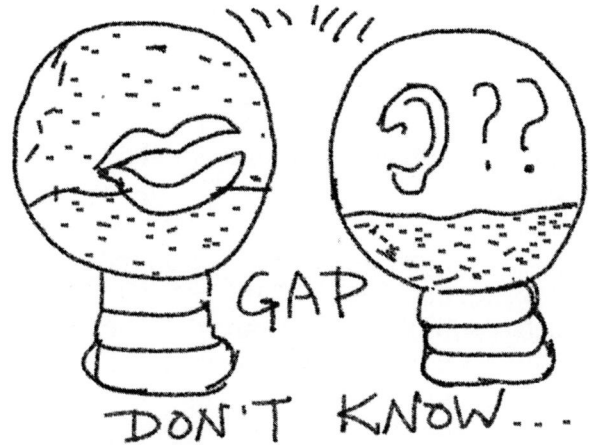

You try to find out what the OTHER person is saying instead of just listening to your own internal talk and opinions about what the other person is saying.

You are completely sincere when you say, "Help me understand what you mean by that."

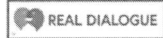

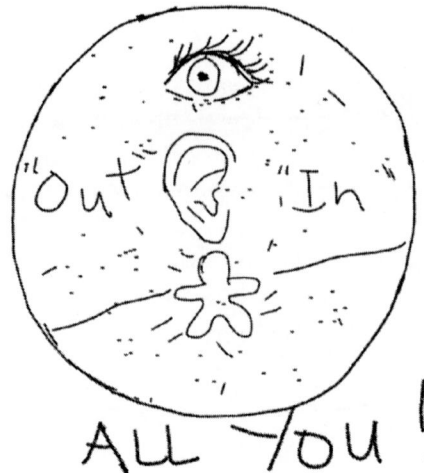

In Speaking for Yourself and Mindful Listening, you develop the muscle to retain a Mindful Gap when you are speaking and listening to others, no matter how upsetting the circumstances and topics are.

First, you speak for yourself, as an individual who cannot read another person's mind.

You remain modest ("I remember it this way") and responsible ("I would like this and I plan to do that.") You stay away from "you-statements" and "we-statements" and "objective facts."

You know the other person is not MAKING you feel a certain way or simply INTERRUPTING you, or simply DISMISSING you.

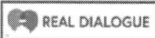

You know the other person has a different snow globe
with a different rhythm and different ears.

You may ask the other person "Are you aware that you
are interrupting me?" And then you try to discover
what is going on: "Help me understand what you are
experiencing right now." You wholly experience that
important boundary between snow globes.

Remember that 100% of what you experience is
subjective, even when you are doing math or learning
objective facts. You process the entire set of what you
experience through your OWN nervous system and it
goes into your cerebral cortex BEFORE you see,
hear or feel it. No one "makes you feel" that way. You
just feel that way.

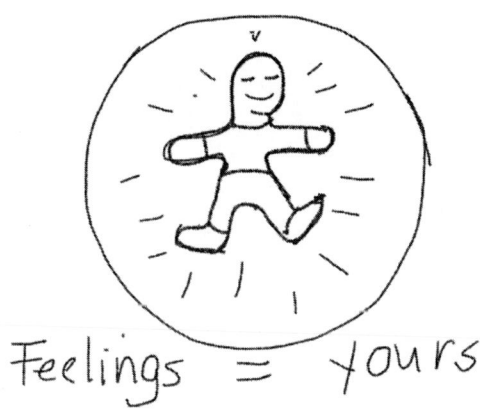

Feelings = yours

Even when we agree about our experience as "reality"
between us, our "shared" experience is still somewhere
between 45% and 85% individual. In other words, we
are guessing at "shared."

 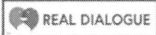

Our lack of consensus only increases when we are emotionally jarred. Our highly subjective "reality" makes us VERY poor eye witnesses. We are unable to agree about what is actually happening much of the time. That's why we argue so much about "what is true" or "what the facts are."

But that doesn't mean you are unaffected by what others say, feel and otherwise express. When someone expresses emotion in a bold or obvious way, you are definitely affected. Emotion that is expressed evokes emotions. Because you are in your own subjective snow globe, though, you cannot know exactly what is evoked in someone else and they cannot know your emotions for certain either, without asking you.

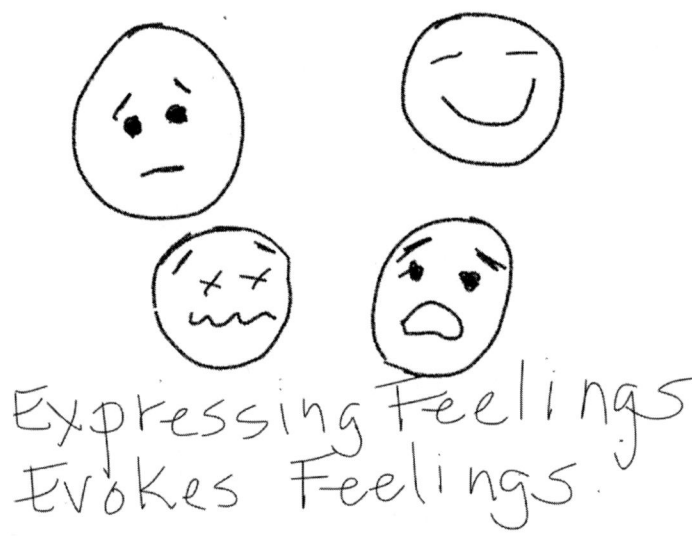

Expressing Feelings Evokes Feelings.

There is no precise hard wiring in adults for what is expressed and what it evokes (for infants and mothers there is more hard wiring). But if humiliation is evoked, a person will likely express rage or simply turn away. For all these reasons, we need to remain curious, even if we think we know what is happening in another snow globe.

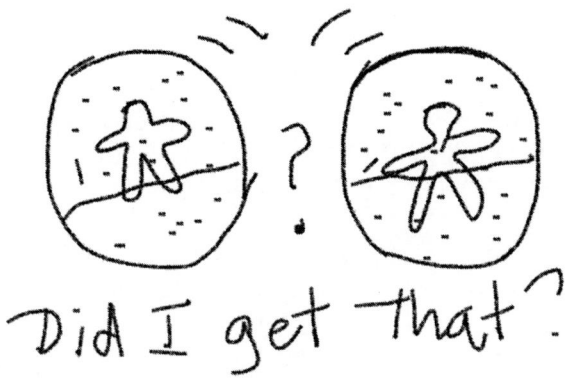

It turns out that the gap between us is the space for love. Maintaining that gap is one of the best things we can do to sustain love with other human beings.

What is love? Mostly it is the continuing warm interest in another person – returning again and again with the desire to know and understand and care. Love is returning again and again to Not-Knowing and the Don't-Know Mind that says "Help me understand what you mean by that." Or "Tell me what it means to feel the way you do."

 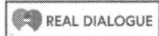

The Mindful Gap makes love go round and round.

When we see how much we do not know, when we understand that we are each enclosed in a subjective space, then we also know we ALL feel alone, set apart, and different from others.

Feeling alone and unknown is not personal; everyone feels it. And that's why warm witnessing and continuing interest are such precious resources.

The Mindful Gap and natural curiosity are generated in Real Dialogue. They invite and allow love to happen, even between people who strongly disagree.

In on-going relationships, we all need to do more than respect each other – although respect is fundamental. We need to see that we need each other in order to understand and witness ourselves.

In difficult conversations, between people who are in the same family, who are in an intimate relationship, or work together on projects over time, Real Dialogue allows us to experience directly how/why we never hear the same thing twice, and how we need curiosity and not judgment each time we come back to our familiar habits in conflict.

The conflicts themselves are not the problem. Being able to see/hear/feel each other, while having the conflicts, is the problem.

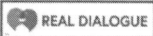

Few of us have the skills to do the seeing/hearing/feeling that is necessary when repetitive conflicts set in. And yet, we all want that kind of witnessing for ourselves. Remaining Curious, when practiced regularly, will almost magically open the door to love - especially in those situations in which you yourself have felt poorly understood or even disrespected.

As you maintain a Mindful Gap and use the skills of Real Dialogue, you will find your way to closer relationships (even during conflicts) and new horizons of meaning at home, at work and in the world.

 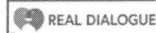

16   The Skill: Volume 3   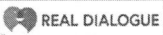 REAL DIALOGUE

Appendix C

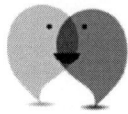

Introduction to Dialogue Therapy
Training

Dialogue Therapy: Designed to Transform Personal Love

- Begins with *falling in love ("just right for me")* – idealizing the beloved and creating an illusion of completion, perfection, of love without hate, of a beloved without flaws

- If it is mutual (two-way street), it develops into power struggles, disillusionment, and the creation of an *Intimate Enemy* who causes one pain, hurt, humiliation, hatred – communicated through projection, identification, projective identification

- Is "taken personally" as in "How can *I* be with someone like *this?*" after disillusionment and projective identification become chronic

- Gives us an opportunity for self-knowledge, wholeness, being able to see, acknowledge, and meet our own needs (through helping ourselves and asking for help)

Dialogue Therapy (DT): What is it?

- Short-term, anxiety-provoking psychoanalytic psychotherapy (STAPP) for couples

- Time-limited to 7 sessions in co-therapist model and 13-14 sessions in solo therapist model (designed originally for co-therapists; see Young-Eisendrath, 1984: pp. 107-158; Young-Eisendrath, 1993/1997)

- Focuses on increased differentiation and intimacy between partners who suffer from repetitive difficulties in resolving conflicts and are enmeshed or emotionally alienated

- Requires commitment to the relationship (including monogamy or the intention to become monogamous), preferably co-habiting

- Relies on a foundation of trust between partners (if trust has been broken, repairing the trust takes place in the first 2 to 3 therapy sessions)

- Fosters direct communication between partners who might otherwise be dependent on the therapist as an intermediary; must deal in session with their conflicts and are not able to triangulate the therapist into the couple (for research on the outcome and process of couple therapy, see for example, Jacobson & Addis, 1993: 85-93)

Sessions of Dialogue Therapy: Co-Therapist Model

1. Introduction, Evaluation, Relational History (3 hours)
2. First Session of DT: Working on a Conflict (2 hours)
3. Second Session: Practicing Skills (2 hours)
4. Third Session: Role Reversal: Empathy for Your Partner (2 hours)
5. Fourth Session: Using Empathy and Dialogue (2 hours)
6. Final Session: Refining Skills (2 hours)
7. Follow-up: Check-in six months later (2 hours)

Room is set up with two chairs facing each other for couple and two chairs slightly behind each partner, out of field of vision. Therapists' chairs (behind) also face each other. Couple receives the brochure about Dialogue Therapy before coming. When all parties are seated, one of the therapists says *"We'd like to hear you talk to each other about why you are here."*

Sessions of Dialogue Therapy: Solo-Therapist Model (all sessions are typically 1 hour):

1. Evaluation and Introduction
2. Evaluation: Relational History of One Partner
3. Evaluation: Relational History of Other Partner
4. First Session of Dialogue Therapy: Working on a Conflict
5. Second Session of Dialogue Therapy: Working on a Conflict
6. Third Session of DT: Practicing Skills
7. Fourth Session of DT: Honing Skills
8. Fifth Session of DT: First Role Reversal – Building Empathy
9. Sixth Session of DT: Second Role Reversal – Building Empathy
10. Seventh Session of DT: Using Empathy and Dialogue
11. Eight Session of DT: Using Empathy and Dialogue
12. Final Session of DT: Refining Skills
13. Follow-up: Check-in six months later

Chairs are set up in the same fashion as co-therapist model.

Methods and Theories: Psychoanalysis

Dialogue Therapy is founded on the psychoanalytic theory of *projective identification* (for definitions see Greenspan & Mannino, 1974: 1103-1106; Modell, 1990: pp. 53-59; Young-Eisendrath 1993/1997: pp. 149-151; Aguayo, 2013: 516-522) as an unconscious or semi-conscious affective communication between partners that disrupts and undermines conscious intentions of individuals and can erode the attachment bond and intimacy over time. When projective identification is *idealizing* (falling in love), it is usually intoxicating for one or both partners. When it transforms into *negativity* or *hostility* during the phase of *disillusionment*, it is painful and deadens the vitality of the relationship.

Dialogue Therapy also draws on psychoanalytic methods of interpreting and finding meaning (for research on the effectiveness of analytic psychotherapy, see, for example, Shedler, 2010) in unconscious affective communication of implied or explicit emotional demands on a partner that originate in an individual's early attachment bonds, relational trauma, or other trauma. (continued on next slide)

Methods and Theories: Psychoanalysis (continued)

These demands lead to "psychological complexes," "repetition compulsions," or implicit "blind spots" (see Banaji & Greenwald, 2016) in an intimate relationship. Partners who come to therapy present their own unique dynamic field of transferences and counter-transferences to each other when they relate, especially on issues that cause threat or conflict.

Dialogue Therapy also draws on Bowlby's attachment model (Bowlby, 1969) as it has been developed in relation to adult pair bonding (see, for example, Ellison & Gray, 2012).

Methods and Theories: Psychodrama

Dialogue Therapy draws on two techniques from psychodrama. (1) "Alter ego" or "doubling": a technique in which a therapist speaks for a partner, using the language and meanings implied by the partner, but saying them in the manner of good dialogue. When there are co-therapists, doubling is done by the co-therapist, who is seated behind and outside the view of one of the partners. The therapist who is the alter ego also interviews that partner in the evaluation session, using the Empathy Interview, and coaches the partner during DT sessions, and sometimes switches chairs with the other partner and does a quick Empathy Interview (later slide) in the midst of failing dialogue. Alter egos (co-therapists) also function as a "reflecting team" in describing and analyzing partner interaction during DT sessions. At some point (third or fourth or later session), DT also incorporates (2) "role reversal" interview in which a partner is asked to "play" the other partner while being interviewed. It's an opportunity to "step into the shoes" of the partner. (For further information, see Blatner, 2000, and Jennings & Holmwood, 2016.)

Methods and Theories: Mindfulness

Dialogue Therapy also draws on mindfulness practices, especially as developed by Shinzen Young (2016) in relation to increasing *concentration, equanimity, and clarity* in everyday life. In order for partners to identify painful blind spots (through projective identification) and overcome a "me" vs. "you" tendency (see Choudhury, 2015, for examples) and to process other emotionally triggering encounters, they have to develop skills in stepping back from active and passive aggression and emotional reactivity. In those moments, they learn to *feel their feelings,* but not express their feelings. Dialogue Therapists give information and short instruction on mindfulness practices and a brief reading (for example, pp. 75-79 from Young, 2016, or pp. 42-45 from Choudhury) as a part of the therapy. Sometimes they may suggest doing mindfulness practice outside of therapy. A partner's ability to *paraphrase* is a good self-assessment of mindfulness skill. Dialogue Therapists should review the evidence base for the effectiveness of mindfulness practices (e.g. Creswell, 2017) and understand some of the ways in which psychoanalytic practices interface with, and differ from, Buddhist practices (e.g. Young-Eisendrath, 2013 and Young-Eisendrath & Dawson, 2008).

Evaluation Session(s)

The evaluation meeting(s) begin with listening to the couple talk to each other about their reasons for coming. After five minutes or so, the co-therapists talk to each other about what they have heard or the solo therapist reflects back to the couple what s/he heard. Then papers and pencils are given to partners and they are asked The Six Questions (next slide).

At the end of this exercise, the answers are read silently by the therapist(s) and the partners are asked to talk with each other about one or more of their answers (depending on what the therapist finds most interesting or revealing). Then, the therapists reflects more on what was heard and any emerging patterns. Then one of the partners is selected for an Empathy Interview: a relational history (later slides). After both partners have been interviewed in this fashion, the therapists pulls up a chair between the partners and offers a "Wrap-Up" or summary of what was discovered in the evaluation. Recommendations for DT or another kind of intervention are made and a short reading assignment is given on the nature of love (selections from Young-Eisendrath, 1993/1997 or Young-Eisendrath, in press).

The Six Questions (Evaluation)

Read aloud to partners with instruction to *"Answer the questions in any way you want. There are no right or wrong answers."*

1. On a scale from 0-10, where zero means *"Take it or leave it"* and 10 means *"As valuable as oxygen,"* How would you rate the value of this relationship for

   you personally?
2. What do you think are the greatest problems in this relationship?
3. What do you think are the greatest benefits in the relationship for you? Why do you stay?
4. How do you think your partner answered the first question?
5. How do you think your partner answered the second question?
6. How do you think your partner answered the third question?

Collect the answers, read them, and ask the couple to talk about one or two.

Empathy Interview

This is a relational history of each partner.

The set-up: For co-therapists, the therapist switches chairs with the partner and faces the person for whom the therapist is the alter ego. Behind the one therapist, seated outside the field of vision, is the co-therapist who will take notes on the interview. Behind the partner being interviewed is the other partner who is also given pen and paper, in case s/he wants to take notes.

Interview begins: *"Let's start with the present moment. Have you noticed an emotional or physical reaction to anything in the session thus far? Anything you want to talk about?"*

Then: *"Please tell me how you look at the problems in this relationship."*
Then: *"OK. I would like to go back to the beginning of your relationship. How did you meet? How old were you? What were the circumstances? Why did you fall in love with X?"*
Then: Trace the development of the relationship, going through major milestones (marriage, children, infidelities, sex, trauma, etc.). (continued on next slide)

Empathy Interview (continued)

When you arrive at the present: *"Have you had other long-term relationships or marriages?"* If so, *"In a nutshell, why did you fall in love and why did you separate?"* (At this point, time management is essential; you have one hour to do this interview, so if there are multiple marriages, you may need to make a choice of how to structure the session.

Eventually you say, *"I want to go back to your family of origin now and get a picture of your mother and father, and then we will talk a little about your siblings. Please start with either parent and give me a picture of how that parent looked to you,–before you were 10 years old."* This is an attempt to get past the narratives we often tell about our parents. If the partner does not answer, return calmly to the instruction: *"Please give me a picture of how your mother/father looked to you. Was s/he tall, short, well-dressed, sloppy? Were you proud or ashamed of her/him?"* After you get a fairly complete answer, then, *"Let's stick with this parent before you were 10 years old: How did you feel with him/her? Could you hug and kiss? Did you climb into her/his lap? Did you say and hear 'I love you'?"* Then ask about anger and criticism. Then ask about favorites among siblings.

Empathy Interview (continued)

Then go forward in time with this parent: *"What was it like after you were 10? In adolescence?"* And then come up to the present and ask about the relationship now. If the parent died, ask about the death. If the death was early in life, ask more details. Ask the same questions about the other parent. If time permits, ask about any grandparents or step-parents who were present a lot in the person's childhood.

Finally, ask about siblings. *"Tell me the sibling order and whether your siblings are married, have children, and have been successful in their lives."*

In the "Wrap-Up," comment especially on the patterns that have obviously carried over from parental relationships to the current relationship. Often, these will be obvious. Remember that these emotional patterns will form the blind spots (Banaji & Greenwald, 2016) or projective-identifications (Young-Eisendrath, 1993/1997: 149–151) that are going to be revealed and overcome through mindfulness and insight in Dialogue Therapy.

Dialogue: A Special Form of Conversation

Dialogue is a form of conversation that allows partners to create a "mindful space" or to "mind the gap" between them (see Young-Eisendrath, 1993/1997 and Young-Eisendrath, 2019). It is a method that is taught and practiced in Dialogue Therapy. Dialogue requires that partners to step back from projective identification and begin to feel and experience their own subjectivity and tendency to "create" the partner as an "intimate enemy" who carries disavowed (especially negative, sometimes idealized) aspects of the self. Dialogue should be used in times of emotionally charged conflict, instead of active aggression (attacking, criticizing) or passive aggression (withdrawing, lying, hiding). The skills of dialogue depend on the ability to incorporate mindfulness and insight into one's emotional habits.

Four Skills of Dialogue

Speaking for Yourself: Using I-statements, staying away from We-statements; formulating your statements in "chunks" short enough for a partner to paraphrase; recognizing the two-way street of back-and-forth; using feeling-oriented formulations when possible (*"I feel [X feeling] when you [do/say/imply/act]"*); not to be slavish to the formula, but to recognize that *perception is subjective.*

Paraphrasing: Summarizing and saying back to your partner what you understand in your own words, if possible; it is not parroting or using a cliché like *"I hear you saying…"*; rather, it requires stepping back from emotional reactivity, being clear about one's feelings, and concentrating on what the other person is trying to communicate; taking responsibility for *what was heard* and not what was said; verifying accuracy at the end of the paraphrase and, if your partner says, "that's not what I meant," trying again until they say "yes, you understood me correctly."

Four Skills of Dialogue (continued)

Being Curious and Expanding the Story: Maintaining a mindful gap means being curious and always trying to get the Big Picture of what your partner is trying to tell you; stepping outside of your own feelings (*Can you feel angry without being angry?*) and seeing if you are able to catch the actual meaning conveyed by the partner; always remaining open to hearing more and expanding the story being conveyed (being empathic does not mean being in agreement)

Responding: After your partner who has concurred that you have understood, then you respond with your own feelings and thoughts in I-statements; you should feel a greater equanimity and clarity after paraphrasing; the sense of a mindful space or gap between you is refreshing and allows for two subjectivities.

Dialogue continues through repeating these four skilled interactions until the conflict is negotiated and resolved or until it is understood and simply allowed to remain a difference between partners. Even in the midst of anger, both partners are respectful and feel respected. Both partners take responsibility for their blind spots.

Projective Identification

An unconscious emotional kidnapping of one person by another person. See Modell (1990), Young-Eisendrath (1993/1997), Young-Eisendrath (2019), and Banaji & Greenwald (2016). The "projector" evokes certain emotional reactions in the other person and the "receiver" then unconsciously plays out what is projected. Often the projection and identification go both ways and both partners feel trapped in a hall of distorting mirrors. *"I am hurt and angry,"* says one and replies the other, *"I am hurt and angry, too."* The unconscious entanglements can be complicated and subtle, based on the mix of unrecognized affective states in the two individuals.

Working on a Conflict: First Session of Dialogue Therapy

Whether using the solo or the co-therapist model, set up the chairs so that partners are facing each other; two "therapist chairs" are placed across from each other and outside the field of vision of couple.

Skills: Alter Ego/Doubling (psychodrama technique), Coaching (leaning in and speaking with a partner about what is disrupting Dialogue), Unblocking (switching chairs with partner and doing short Empathy Interview)

Beginning: *I would like to hear the two of you talk about what you would like to focus on for this session. We will be using the skills of Dialogue as they are described in Chapter 4 of "Love Between Equals" (assigned before this session). Briefly describe: Speaking for Yourself, Paraphrasing, Responding, Expanding Curiosity.*

Wait for partners to decide on what they want to talk about and help them *only* if they begin to be actively or passively aggressive. Stop the aggression and coach the partner on Speaking for Yourself

Working on a Conflict: First Session of Dialogue Therapy (continued)

After the topic is chosen, say this: *One of you can begin speaking and the other person will need to paraphrase; check on whether the statement is understood before responding. I will help you with this process by using the techniques of Alter Ego or Doubling and Coaching.* (In the co-therapist model, I will also consult with my co-therapist from time to time.)

When I am speaking as your alter ego, I will speak as though I am you. I will keep my eyes down and not look up at your partner. I will speak over your shoulder. If you agree that the words express what you are experiencing, let them stand, and your partner can respond to them as though you were saying them. If you want to tweak my words or change them, feel free to do that.

When I am coaching you, I will lean forward and use your name, look at you, and coach you or ask you what is going on with you. When coaching you, I may ask to change seats with your partner and speak to you briefly about the issues that are creating obstacles in you being able to use Dialogue.

After the couple has chosen the topic, have them begin.

Working on a Conflict: First Session of Dialogue Therapy (continued)

In the initial session of Working on a Conflict, you will have to intervene frequently with coaching, doubling and unblocking.

Wrap-up comes at the end of the session with the chairs pulled into a circle. You share your understanding, use the skills of dialogue, and send the couple out with something to read or something to do. You might assign chapters of *Love Between Equals* and/or ask them to practice Dialogue skills. If they are unable to contain emotional distress in practicing the skills, do not ask them to practice at home. Give them some reading instead.

Working on a Conflict: Practicing Skills, Honing Skills of Dialogue

In all following DT sessions, you help the couple practice the skills of Dialogue, integrating the themes that were discovered in the Evaluation sessions, in order to break up the projective identification and open a space for Mindful Witnessing and Differentiation.

The therapeutic techniques used by the Dialogue Therapist will be Doubling/Alter Ego, Coaching, Unblocking. In the unblocking you work to help the individual understand the themes of the projective identification for that individual and to manage/contain the emotional agitation in order to be able to listen to the partner and begin to find curiosity and respect during conflict with the partner.

Each session begins with exactly the same directive as the first session of DT: *I would like to hear the two of you talk about what you would like to focus on in this session.* You use the directive in ALL subsequent DT sessions.

There is a designated number of sessions for the co-therapist and solo models. You try to stick to that number of sessions. If you have to modify, you add one or two sessions (whether to the Evaluation or the subsequent sessions). This is time-limited therapy. You expect the couple to improve in using the skills of Dialogue. If this is not happening, you tell them repeatedly during the coaching that they are responsible for learning the skills and that the therapy will not help them unless they use the skills at home.

Idealization

Idealization is a fanciful or fantasy love that can never be sustained over time because it is not based on the reality of another person and makes conflict impossible (Young-Eisendrath, 2008, pp. 174-79). Idealizing a person means that you see him or her as "perfect" or as being just want you want, desire, need, or deserve to "complete" you or protect or enhance you. Idealization creates an "object of desire" and does not perceive a real person. Parents idealize their children, children idealize their parents, romance demands idealization, romantic comedy feeds on idealization, and pornography creates idealized objects that can be controlled. Idealization always leads to disillusionment because human beings are limited, imperfect, and changing. They cannot be perfected.

Anger not Aggression

Anger: The feeling of indignation based on a perceived injustice or unfairness or hurt. The Greeks called anger "the moral emotion" because they observed human beings using anger to right injustice, but they saw that animals could not do such a thing. Whereas animals could only use the aggression of fight or flee, humans had another choice. (For a fuller analysis, see Travis, 1989.) They could *reflect* on their situation and create a boundary against injustice instead of fighting or retreating. Used skillfully, anger is a boundary-setting emotion. It is not an attack or a withdrawal. It is an I-state of *"I am angry because…"* or *"I won't tolerate this because…"* or *"I don't like this because…"* It is not a You-statement. When anger is used effectively, partners can communicate their boundaries and their hurts, often leading to greater intimacy.

Anger not Aggression (continued)

Aggression: an instinctual response to threat or fear; it is technically not an emotion, but an innate reactivity of the limbic system that causes fight (blame, criticize, attack, trivialize) or flee (withhold, stonewall, procrastinate, turn aggression against the self). Aggression begets aggression and erodes trust. (For a review of active and passive aggression, see pp. 14-15 in Wiley & Kite, 2013.)

Separation Anxiety

The instinctual response to a "separation threat" or to an actual unwanted separation from a loved one with whom one has a bond (see Bowlby, 1973). Experienced as restlessness, anxiety, and checking behavior, you may cycle repeatedly through rage, depression, and apathy (indifference). Separation anxiety may occur through feelings of wanting to leave a committed relationship, coming from oneself, but is always stirred up when one or both partners make threats of leaving.

Building Empathy for Self and Partner: Role Reversal

This intervention will take two hours, whether using the solo or co-therapist model, it's 30 minutes of role reversal with a partner, and then some dialogue about the effects on the partner, and observations of what was seen and heard, and then repeated with the other partner, followed by some dialogue. If done in two one hour meetings, there will be a Wrap-up at the end of each.

After the opening (listening to couple deciding on the topic), you can listen to more dialogue and see what is developing or you can switch chairs immediately. Listening to the couple's dialogue might help you know when to intervene with Role Reversal.

Switch chairs with the partner and sit across from the interviewee and say: *This interview is called a Role Reversal and it gives us an opportunity to see your empathy for your partner, to see how accurately you perceive your partner. I am going to interview you as though you were you partner, using your partner's name. You do not have to act or sound like your partner, although you can do that if you would like, but I would like you to step into your partner's shoes and answer the questions as you think your partner would.* Then you begin the interview, often picking up a thread from what the couple was just talking about. Ask questions that arise from your curiosity and what the partners are talking about and then ask the standard questions from the next slide. You will always ask the standard questions.

Building Empathy for Self and Partner: Role Reversal (continued)

If you had a magic wand and could change one thing about yourself X, what would it be?

Same question about partner – explore the answers.

What do you like best/most about yourself, X?

What do you like best/most about your partner, X?

How do you feel about your sex life with your partner, X?

How do you feel about your partner as a parent? (if the person has children)?

Where do you want to be five years from now in this relationship?

After each empathy interview, have the partner come back and offer feedback and reflections.

Wrap-up at the end of the hour.

Contraindications for Dialogue Therapy

The evaluation session should be used as assessment and no contract should be made with a couple until the evaluation is complete. It is essential to assess for active addictions, violence, infidelity, separation, and personality disorders. In general, couples should not engage in DT when there is active violence or substance abuse that is untreated. Individuals should be referred for treatment and invited to come back for DT when they are in treatment. If there is an active infidelity, DT is usually effective unless the unfaithful partner is not willing to commit to the primary relationship. *"If you want to come to DT you need to give up the outside relationship and be willing to repair the trust with your partner."*) This usually means that the first two or three meetings of DT are focused on repairing trust. DT is not effective for separating couples. If partners are not both fully committed to the relationship, then individual psychotherapy should be recommended because choosing to be in or out of a relationship is an individual choice. Borderline and narcissistic personality disorders can be hard to manage in the structured set-up of DT (Consult the The Psychodynamic Diagnostic Manual, 2006, or its 2nd edition, in press, for descriptions of personality disorders)

Bibliography for the Introduction to Dialogue Therapy

Aguayo, J. (2013). Review of *Projective identification: The fate of a concept. Psychoanalytic Psychology, 30,* 516-522.

Banaji, M. & Greenwald, A. (2016). *Blind spot: Hidden biases of good people.* NY: Bantam.

Blatner, A. (2000). *Foundations of psychodrama: History, theory, and practice (4th edition).* NY: Springer.

Bowlby, J. (1969). *Attachment and loss: Vol. 1.* London, Eng: Hogarth Press.

Bowlby, J. (1973). *Attachment and loss: Separation: Vol. 2.* London, Eng: Hogarth Press.

Catherall, D. (1992). Working with projective identification in couples. *Family Process,* 31:4, 355-367.

Choudhury, S. (2015). *Deep diversity: Overcoming us vs. them.* Toronto, ON: Between the Lines.

Coontz, S. (2006). *Marriage, a history: How love conquered marriage.* NY: Penguin.

Creswell, J.D. (2017). Mindfulness interventions. *Annual Review of Psychology,* 68:1, 419-516.

Ellison, P. & Gray, P. (Eds.) (2012). Endrocrinology of social relationships. Cambridge, MA: Harvard University Press.

Bibliography for the Introduction to Dialogue Therapy

Greenspan, S. & Mannino, F. (1974). A model for brief intervention with couples based on projective identification. *American Journal of Psychiatry, 131*:10, 1103-1106.

Jacobson, N. & Addis, M. (1993). Research on couples and couples therapy: What do we know? Where are we going? *Journal of Consulting and Clinical Psychology, 61*:1, 85-93.

Jennings, S. & Holmwood, C. (2016). *Routledge handbook of psychodrama.* Abingdon, Eng: Routledge.

Modell, A. (1990). *Other times, other realities: Toward a theory of psychoanalytic treatment.* Cambridge, MA: Harvard University Press.

PDM Task Force. (2006). *Psychodynamic diagnostic manual.* Silver Spring, MD: Alliance of Psychoanalytic Organizations.

Shedler, J. (2010). The efficacy of psychodynamic psychotherapy. *American Psychologist, 65*:2, 98-109.

Travis, C. (1989). *Anger: The misunderstood emotion.* NY: Simon & Schuster/Touchstone.

Wiley, B. & Kite, M. (2013). *Principles of research in behavioral science (3rd Edition).* NY: Routledge.

Young, S. (2016). *The science of enlightenment: How meditation works.* Boulder, CO: Sounds True.

Bibliography for the Introduction to Dialogue Therapy

Young-Eisendrath, P. (1984). *Hags and heroes: A feminist approach to Jungian psychotherapy with couples.* Toronto, ON: Inner City Books.

Young-Eisendrath, P. (1993/1997). *You're not what I expected: Love after the romance has ended.* NY: William Morrow/Fromm International.

Young-Eisendrath, P. (2008). *The self-esteem trap: Raising confident and compassionate kids in an age of self-importance.* NY: Little Brown.

Young-Eisendrath, P. (2008). Jung and Buddhism: Refining the dialogue. In P. Young-Eisendrath & T. Dawson (Eds.), *The Cambridge Companion to Jung (2nd Edition).* Cambridge, Eng: Cambridge University Press.

Young-Eisendrath, P. (2013). Introduction. In P. Young-Eisendrath (Ed.), *Buddhism and depth psychology: Refining the encounter, Spring Journal,* 89, 1-14.

Young-Eisendrath, P. (2014). *The present heart: A memoir of love, loss and discovery.* NY: Rodale.

Young-Eisendrath, P. (2019). *Love between equals: Relationship as a spiritual path.* Boulder, CO: Shambhala Publications.

Appendix D

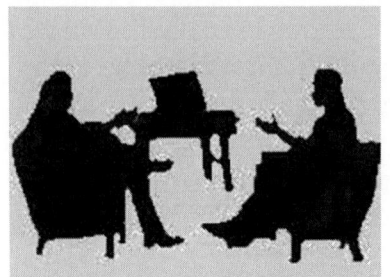

Index

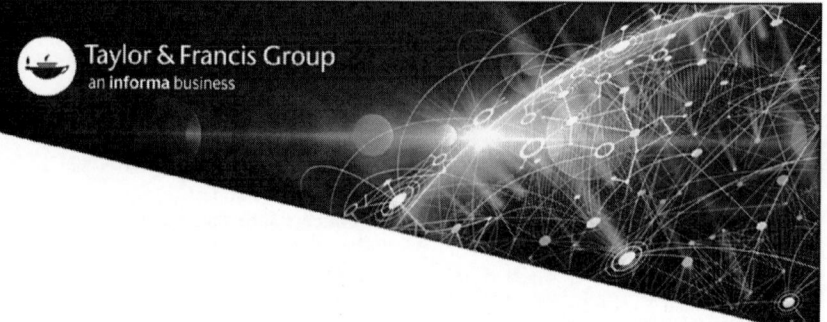
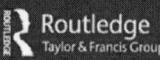
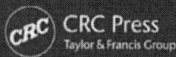